To my Good friend
DAVE SANDERS
with Best Wishes
for a continued
success in
Medical Devices

IMPLANTS
Reconstructing the Human Body

IMPLANTS

Reconstructing the Human Body

Wilfred Lynch

VAN NOSTRAND REINHOLD COMPANY
NEW YORK CINCINNATI TORONTO LONDON MELBOURNE

Copyright © 1982 by Van Nostrand Reinhold Company Inc.

Library of Congress Catalog Card Number: 81-16138
ISBN: 0-442-24968-3

Manufactured in the United States of America

Published by Van Nostrand Reinhold Company Inc.
135 West 50th Street, New York, N.Y. 10020

Van Nostrand Reinhold Publishing
1410 Birchmount Road
Scarborough, Ontario MIP 2E7, Canada

Van Nostrand Reinhold Australia Pty. Ltd.
17 Queen Street
Mitcham, Victoria 3132, Australia

Van Nostrand Reinhold Company Limited
Molly Millars Lane
Wokingham, Berkshire, England

15   14   13   12   11   10   9   8   7   6   5   4   3   2   1

Library of Congress Cataloging in Publication Data

Lynch, Wilfred.
  Implants: Reconstructing the Human Body

  Includes index.
  1. Prosthesis. I. Title. [DNLM: 1. Artificial
organs. 2. Implants, Artificial. 3. Prosthesis,
WO 176 L987m]
RD130.L86   617′95′0028   81-16138
ISBN 0-442-24968-3   AACR2

To my wife Candace
who edited and typed the manuscript and had to organize the
material despite my irregular schedule of writing.

W.L.

Preface

The human body is an assembly of remarkable biomechanisms ingeniously integrated and incorporating design features which cannot be duplicated as well or as compactly by our current engineering knowledge. There are, however, a growing number of effective artificial organs being manufactured on a production line basis. These modern prosthetic devices can add years to an individual's useful life, improve physical comfort, or in the case of aesthetic implants, improve emotional stability.

Because of the increased popular interest in "spare body parts," this book is intended as a general introduction to this fascinating field. It is aimed to the medical student, biomedical engineer, and physician, who would like to keep up with the latest developments in prosthetics. The language is complicated as little as possible with medical terminology; consequently, it can be understood by interested nonmedical technical people and by the inquisitive layman.

Emphasis is placed upon the design and function of devices from an engineering point of view. The anatomy and physiology of body functions are presented in whatever detail deemed necessary to support an understanding of the function of the specific device. Sometimes a substantial advance in surgical procedure has had to be made prior to the routine use of a prosthetic device. One example is the bypass of the heart and lungs with extracorporeal circulation through a "heart-lung" machine prior to the replacement of a diseased heart valve. Such procedures are also described.

The ultimate success of a prosthetic implant depends a great deal on the materials used in its construction. Very few materials have the combination of properties which allow them to survive in the hostile environment of the body and at the same time prove to be nontoxic. Currently used and promising new developmental materials are discussed in Chapter 1 along with the tests commonly required to determine their suitability in biomedical applications.

There has been no attempt to cover dental and maxillofacial prosthetics. This is such a large and important field it warrants a book by itself. Development of modern prosthetic materials started, in many cases, with the dental specialty: the chromium cobalt alloys used in joint applications today were first applied in partial dentures and the success of acrylic denture base material led to its use as surgical bone cement.

WILFRED LYNCH

Contents

Preface   vii

1. MATERIALS   1
Polymeric Materials for Implants   4
A Natural Polymer   15
Metals   16
Ceramics   18
Safety Testing of Implant Materials   19

2. SKELETON AND JOINT PROSTHESES   24
Joints   26
Implants for Orthotics   44

3. CARDIOVASCULAR IMPLANTS   48
Valves   53

4. DEVICES IN UROLOGY   95

**5. IMPLANTS FOR THE IMPROVEMENT OF SEXUAL
FUNCTION**   107

6. IMPLANTS FOR VISION, HEARING, AND VOICE   120
Anatomy and Physiology of the Eye   120
The Ear   133
Voice Restoration after Laryngectomy   141

7. IMPLANTS FOR AESTHETIC SURGERY   148

8. NEUROLOGICAL IMPLANTS   168
The Brain, the Nervous System, and Electroneural Stimulation   168

Glossary   189

Index   199

IMPLANTS
Reconstructing the Human Body

1
Materials

Modern materials and the knowledge of their fabrication represent the real keystone of the success and rapid growth in the use of implants over the last two decades. Ingenious design engineering, coupled with skillful surgery, naturally played a great part in this achievement; however, the development of dependable surgical implants proceeded at a snail's pace until the emergence of "exotic" new materials in answer to the needs of the military in World War II. The subsequent aerospace program and the high volume demands of burgeoning new postwar industries made the commercial production of these unique materials practical.

Man-made materials cannot, given the current state of the art, duplicate the characteristics of the structures which make up the human body. Very few synthetic materials exhibit physical properties comparable to those of human tissue or have the ability to withstand as well the hostile environment of the body for a prolonged period. The few materials which do must also prove to be nontoxic and noncarcinogenic.

The extensive testing (presented at the end of this chapter) currently required to prove an acceptable level of biocompatibility for a new material is so time consuming and expensive that the choice of implant materials increases very slowly.

The implant materials in popular use may be broadly classified as polymers, metals, and ceramics. Polymers would include plastics, rubbers, gels, and fluids.

Polymers are large, long chain molecules synthesized from simple molecules called monomers. An example of a plastic polymer which is common in household articles such as milk, freezer, and other storage containers, and is also used as an implant material, is polyethylene. Polyethylene is made by the polymerization (synthesis) of the simple organic compound ethylene. Many thousands of ethylene molecules are joined together to form polyethylene.

Ethylene

becomes

This polyethylene chain could typically contain 150,000 carbon atoms and be 18 μm long (.0006 inch); at the scale used in the diagram, it would extend over more pages than this entire book.

It is convenient for the chemist to depict the structure of polymer molecules as being straight and rigid, and to picture them all lying in neat rows alongside each other. However, if we were to magnify a polymer until individual molecules became visible, it would more likely resemble a plate of spaghetti all intertwined and folded back and forth. Polyethylene is referred to as *thermoplastic* because it softens on heating and can be formed into a shape which will be retained on cooling. On reheating, it will soften and can be reshaped. Chemical cross-linking of the polymer chains in such a way that they are all joined together in a three dimensional network, produces a *thermosetting* polymer. Thermosetting polymers do not soften on heating, so the cross-linking (also called vulcanization) must occur after the polymer is shaped by the molding or extrusion process. Thermosetting polymers are also insoluble, although swelling can occur when they are exposed to organic solvents. The key properties of polymeric materials may be found in Table 1-1.

Table 1-1. Comparison of Properties of Implant Materials

	STIFFNESS		TENSILE STRENGTH		OUTSTANDING CHARACTERISTICS
	psi $\times 10^5$	GP$_a$	psi $\times 10^3$	MP$_a$	
ELASTOMERS					
Silicone	.58	.4	.8–1.2	5.5–8.3	Soft, non-deteriorating
Bion™			1.8–2.5	12–17	Exceptional flex life
Urethane			2–8.4	13.8–58	Strong, abrasion resistant
PLASTICS					
Teflon			2–5	13.8–34.5	Inert
UHMW polyethylene	.2–1.1	.14–.76	5.6–6.4	38.6–44	Lowest coefficient of friction, high wear resistance
Polysulfone	3.6	2.48	10.3	71	Strong, stiffness close to bone
Acrylic	3.8–4.5	2.6–3.1	7–11	48–75.8	Retention of clarity
Polyester	4.6–6	3.17–4.1	8.5–10.5	58.6–72	Strong, non-deteriorating fibers
BONE					
Cancellous	1–7	.69–4.8	12	82.7	Ideal combination of strength, resilience and lightweight
Cortical	10–30	6.9–20.7	18	124	
METALS					
Titanium alloy	160	110	146	1006	Corrosion resistence, lightweight
316 Stainless steel	290	200	140	965	Easily fabricated
Chromium cobalt alloy	330	227	155	1068	Wear resistant
CARBON					
Pyrolitic	25–45	17–31	7	48	Wear resistant, unique tissue compatability
Fiber	377–580	260–400	290–435	2000–3000	Highest strength, unique tissue compatability

The materials are listed in increasing order of stiffness (tensile modulus) since this is an important physical characteristic when attempting to match the variety of human tissues.

POLYMERIC MATERIALS FOR IMPLANTS

Acrylics

The thermoplastic polymethyl methacrylate

$$\left[-CH_2-\underset{\underset{CO_2CH_3}{|}}{\overset{\overset{CH_3}{|}}{C}}- \right]_n$$

better known by the trade names Plexiglas* and Lucite†, is very stable
and well tolerated by the body. Because of its clarity, it is often used as a
lens implant in the eye after cataract surgery, and because it is easily
formed and colored, it is used for the manufacture of very realistic
looking artificial eyeballs.

Polymethyl methacrylate powder, when mixed with approximately
30% liquid methyl methacrylate monomer containing a small amount
of initiator, forms a dough-like mass which can be easily shaped. In
5–10 minutes after mixing, the material hardens, accompanied by a
considerable release of heat. This type of self-curing acrylic cement was
initially used in dentistry as a denture base, liner, and repair material. It
is now the most commonly used bone cement in orthopedic surgery.

As a bone cement the product is mixed and applied at the time of
insertion of the prosthesis. During mixing and molding into the bone
cavity, there is some loss of the monomer component. The monomer is
quite toxic—the most common and severe effect being transient
lowering of the blood pressure.[1] Cases of cardiac arrest associated with
the use of acrylic bone cement have been reported. Therefore, care
must be taken by the surgeon to mix the cement thoroughly and to
minimize its contact with adjacent tissues when inserting it into the
bone cavity. There is no adhesion of acrylic bone cement to either bone
or prosthetic implant; its holding power is strictly a result of
mechanical locking. Consequently, it can be loosened if subjected to
the shock of anything but low level patient activity. The exotherm is
vigorous enough to reach temperatures approaching $> 70°C$, a temperature which could cause some necrosis of adjoining bone tissue.[2]

---

*Rohm & Haas. Philadelphia, PA.
† Du Pont, Wilmington, DE.

The popularity of acrylic bone cement, despite these problems, lies in its speed and ease of handling. Much research effort is being spent on alternatives. As yet, none have proved as acceptable.

A hydrophilic acrylic polymer, poly-2-hydroxyethyl methacrylate, which is completely compatible with human tissue, has been successfully used as a soft contact lens.*

Polyethylene

Polyethylene is a thermoplastic polymer which is so well tolerated when implanted in vivo that it is used as a standard of comparison in the toxicity testing of biomaterials. It is resistant to all acids, alkalis, and inorganic chemicals and is insoluble at room temperature. It has a very low coefficient of friction and outstanding wear resistance. Consequently, the ultra high molecular weight (UHMW)† polyethylene, which is the strongest type, is used for articulation surfaces in joints. Some of the UHMW polyethylene joint parts are further reinforced by the incorporation of carbon fibers (see "composites").

Other applications include otological implants and mesh‡ used in repairs of the chest wall and diaphragm. Porous high density polyethylene, which in animal studies readily accepts the ingrowth of bone and soft tissue, is being tested clinically as a bond coating for joint prostheses: it is also used in implants for otology.

Polytetrafluoroethylene§

Direct reaction between polyethylene and fluorine will convert the polyethylene to polytetrafluoroethylene (PTFE). The carbon chain becomes completely saturated with fluorine atoms:

---

*Soflens—Bausch & Lomb, Inc., Rochester, NY.
†The most serviceable combination of physical properties appears to accompany a molecular weight 2×10^6.
‡Marlex-Phillips. Chemical Co., Bartlesville, Okla.
§ *Teflon—Du Pont, Wilmington, DE.*

PTFE conforms to the structure of a thermoplastic polymer, but its molecular weight and crystallinity are so high that it cannot be fabricated by the molding or extrusion processes generally applied to thermoplastic materials. PTFE must be processed by sintering, which is the compacting of fine powder under very high temperatures and pressures. It is probably the most inert of the plastic materials and it has the lowest coefficient of friction. Despite these attributes, its use in the body is quite limited because of poor physical properties— particularly its tendency to cold flow.

In an expanded, reinforced form* it is used as a blood vessel replacement, and small quantities are used for otology protheses. Powdered PTFE mixed to a paste consistency with glycerin† has been injected, with satisfactory results, into the larynx to improve phonation in the case of unilateral vocal cord paralysis.

Fluorocarbon Fluid—Artificial Blood

Perfluorodecalin,

a fluorocarbon fluid which can dissolve and transport tremendous amounts of oxygen, has been used successfully as a blood substitute in Japan.

Known as Fluosol‡-DA, the artificial blood promises to be a great boon where rare types such as O negative may not be regularly available on the battlefield or at the scene of accidents.

The fluorocarbon, as a stable emulsion, is injected into the blood stream where is performs the oxygen carrying function of the red blood cells until the body has replenished its own supply of cells. Fluosol has no apparent tissue reaction. It is not metabolized but is gradually eliminated from the body. Over a dozen American and more than 200 persons in Japan had received the blood substitute by 1980.[3]

---

* Gore-tex—W. L. Gore & Assoc., Inc., Elkton, MD.
† Polytef PTFE—Mentor Division, Codman & Shurtleff, Inc., Randolph, MA.
‡ The Green Cross Pharmaceutical Co., Osaka, Japan (Dr. Ryoichi Naito).

Polyester

The polyester, polyethylene terephthalate,

$$\left[\begin{array}{c} \overset{O}{\overset{\|}{C}}\text{—}\bigcirc\text{—}\overset{O}{\overset{\|}{C}}OCH_2CH_2O \end{array}\right]_n$$

is produced as a fiber* which is used to make a variety of fabrics used as implants. Its widest use is probably in knit arterial prostheses. Felt and open weave polyesters have been used as stroma on silicone and other implants to permit tissue fixation. While polyester is quite stable as an implant material, it does cause more tissue reaction than other implant materials, thereby encouraging the growth of tissue into open weave structures and promoting quick fixation. Polyester mesh is used to reinforce silicone rubber sheet used in a variety of surgical reconstructive procedures. The monofilament form is used in the manufacture of strong nonabsorbable sutures—the suture surface is usually treated with Teflon or silicone.

Polysulfones

Sulfone polymers are rigid, transparent, thermoplastics which are exceptionally strong, tough, and resistant to high temperatures:

$$\left[\bigcirc\text{—}O\text{—}\bigcirc\text{—}\overset{O}{\overset{\|}{\underset{\underset{O}{\|}}{S}}}\right]_n$$

They can be fabricated to very close tolerances and can be steam autoclaved repeatedly. Small quantities of relatively new medical grade polysulfones† have been used in heart valve and pacer components as well as in neurological implants. However, much larger volumes are used in medical instrumentation applications.

The use of porous polysulfone as a bone implant material has been

---

*Dacron—Du Pont, Wilmint, DE, Terylene—Imperial Chemical Industries.
† Udel—Union Carbide Corporation, New York, N.Y.

studied.[4] Observations indicate ideal mechanical properties and satisfactory bone growth into the polysulfone. In polysulfones produced by
sintering, the interconnecting porosity exhibited openings of 40–400
μm. The modulus of elasticity was several times higher than porous
UHMW polyethylene and the tensile strength about double.

Polyurethane Elastomer

Polyurethane is a generic term applied to the literally hundreds of
different compounds resulting from the reaction of a diisocyanate
(OCN—R—NCO) with a polyol (HO—R—OH). Noted for their high
strength, abrasion and tear resistance, and versatility of fabrication,
the early urethanes demonstrated a relatively high degree of bio-
degradability and, consequently, after some initial trials were avoided
as implant materials.

Recent advances involving new diisocyanate/polyol/additive combinations have led to great resistance to hydrolysis and excellent flex
life. Figure 3-29 illustrates the application of the improved polyurethane in a critical implant application—the insulation of an
intravenous lead for a heart pacemaker.

Silicones

Silicone is a popular term used to describe a whole family of
organosilicon polymers based on a backbone or molecular chain of
alternate silicon and oxygen atoms:

$$\cdots\underset{\underset{CH_3}{|}}{\overset{\overset{CH_3}{|}}{Si}}-O-\underset{\underset{CH_3}{|}}{\overset{\overset{CH_3}{|}}{Si}}-O-\underset{\underset{CH_3}{|}}{\overset{\overset{CH_3}{|}}{Si}}-O\cdots$$

Dimethyl polysolixane

Depending on the length of the chain and the organic groups attached
to the silicon atoms, these compounds range all the way from water-
thin through heavy oil-like fluids to greases, gels, rubbers, and solid
resins.

The silicones are exceptionally stable and higly biocompatible. The
bioacceptability of the silicones is supported by a great volume of
research. Even the fluids are stable. They do not break down in the

animal body environment, and it is well established that medical grade silicones do no physiological harm. Detailed animal studies may be found in reports by Rowe,[5] Child,[6] and Paul[7] in which ingestion of silicone fluids over long periods of time revealed no differences between experimental and control groups in growth, hematology, bone marrow, organ weights, and histopathology. It is interesting to note that similar amounts of mineral oil fed to rats did cause a connective tissue response in liver and spleen. Also, in the case of the observations of Paul, at least 96% of the fluid ingested was recovered from the feces and gastrointestional tract. Little response was noted when pure grades of silicone fluids were injected subcutaneously, intramuscularly, or into the vitreous cavity of the eye. Silicone fluids injected subcutaneously are being used under FDA supervision to treat facial hemiatrophy (Romberg's disease). Silicones are not attacked by microorganisms. Lack of reproductive, teratologic, and mutagenic response has been reported by Hobbs.[8] A clean bill of health is given to silicones regarding potential environmental damage; it has been shown that silicones do not accumulate in the flesh or eggs of chickens, or in fish.

Silicone rubber is the material of choice for soft tissue restoration in plastic surgery. Tens of thousands of "acute series tests" based on United States Pharmacopeia procedures have proved its nontoxic nature. However, the most convincing evidence of all is the experience plastic surgeons have had with their patients. Over a period of more than 20 years there have been no apparent silicone rubber implant related carcinomas or other serious side effects.

Silicone rubber, a thermosetting elastomer produced by the crosslinking of high molecular weight silicone gums, is the most versatile of all elastomers:

It can be produced over a broad range of hardness and modulus without the addition of plasticizers; nor does it need antioxidants, ultraviolet absorbers, or the many additives which are regularly mixed with other elastomers and which reduce their biocompatibility.

Silicone rubber can be easily fabricated into a variety of tubes and molded shapes[9] which, because of high thermal stability, can be sterilized repeatedly by steam or even dry heat.

The applications for implant grades of silicone rubber include prostheses for ophthalmology, otology, neurology, laryngology, esophagology, facial reconstruction, breast augmentation and reconstruction, augmentation and reconstruction of the genitalia, urinary conduit reconstruction, finger, toe, and wrist joint replacement, and tendon replacement. Also incorporating silicone rubber are implantable heart pacer leads and power source, neurostimulator leads and loop antennae, drug release capsules, etc.

Silicones can be copolymerized with urethanes, styrenes, carbonates, and other chemical groups to form polymers exhibiting some desirable features of both. An example is Avcothane 51* elastomer, a block copolymer of 10% poly(dialkyl siloxane) and 90% poly(ether urethane). This material is both strong (tensile strength as high as 6000 psi) and highly hemocompatible. It has been used with record success for the fabrication of intra-aortic ballon pumps.

A Polyolefin Elastomer

An elastomeric polymer which, along with all the other attributes of a good biomaterial, can withstand rigorous continued flexing with practically no deterioration has long been sought for use in finger and other joints, artificial heart components, and the like.

Bion† is a stereoregular synthetic elastomer prepared from unsaturated mono-olefin and 4/5-methyl-1,4-hexadiene. Exceptional flex-fatigue characteristics are realized‡, probably resulting in large part from the fully saturated backbone and the self-plasticizing nature of the pendant alkyl chains.

---

*Trademark, Avco-Everett Co., Everett, MA.
†Trademark, Lord Corporation, Erie, PA.
‡ Specimens subjected to the DeMattia flex tester are still on test after over 300×10^6 cycles; for other properties see Table 1-I.

$$\begin{array}{c} CH_3 \quad CH_3 \\ \diagdown \quad \diagup \\ C \\ \| \\ CH \\ | \\ CH_2 \end{array}$$

Relatively new on the implant scene, Bion has been used clinically only in the production of finger joints (see Chapter 2) but promises wide application wherever long flex life and good damping characteristics are required.

Carbon

Carbon occurs in a number of forms displaying an extraordinarily wide range of properties, including a unique immunity from fatigue. Some forms of carbon exhibit outstanding biocompatibility and are being used increasingly as a tissue interface in a variety of implant applications. (Carbon is introduced here along with the polymers, although it is not usually considered one,* because high strength carbon fibers are being effectively used as reinforcement of composite implant materials.)

Carbon Fibers. Carbon fibers are made by the pyrolization of polymer fibers such as polyacrylonitrile or rayon at very high temperatures, in an inert atmosphere. Depending on the chemical, mechanical, and thermal history of the fibers during processing, they can be produced in a wide range of stiffness, and their ultimate tensile strength can run as high as 3 GPa (435000 psi). They can be felted, woven into cloth, or used as monodirectional filaments when applied as composite reinforcements. Besides their use in composites, carbon fibers have been successfully used as tendon- and ligament-forming implants.[11]

---

*The term *polymeric carbon* has been used by Jenkins and Kawamura[10] to describe the polyaromatic ribbon structure of fibrous and vitreous carbons.

Vitreous Carbon. Another form of polymeric carbon—vitreous or glassy carbon—may be prepared by the pyrolysis of a machined or molded polymer shape, in an inert atmosphere, at about 1800°C. Despite its excellent biocompatibility and ease of production in various configurations, its low impact strength and high notch sensitivity leave much to be desired for its use as a practical implant material. However, carbon-fiber-reinforced vitreous carbon shows considerable promise for a variety of implants (see "Composites").

Pyrolytic carbon is an isotropic form deposited at high temperatures when a pure hydrocarbon gas is thermally cracked. It may be deposited on a premachined substrate of any material which can withstand the particular process temperature. When cracking is carried out on the low side of the possible temperature range, the result is a higher strength product. So-called low temperature isotropic (LTI) pyrolitic carbon is processed at about 1300°C (2372°F). Consequently, graphite is usually used as the substrate material. The thin LTI coating which is deposited in a fluidized bed process, is strong, hard, and fracture resistant.* It can be made stronger and very wear resistant by alloying with 8–15 wt% of silicon. This is accomplished by the introduction of methyltrichlorosilane[12] (CH_3SiCl_3) to the hydrocarbon gas during the pyrolitic cracking. Small silicon particles are formed and codeposited with the carbon.

Outstanding in its compatibility with blood and exhibiting remarkable toughness and wear resistance, LTI pyrolitic carbon has been used successfully in hundreds of thousands of heart valve components without a failure resulting from the carbon coating.[12] Pyrolitic carbon also shows promise for use in joint articulation surfaces.

Carbon actively promotes new tissue growth[13] and when a microporous carbon surface is presented, the tissue will bond to the interface. Consequently, although there is still much clinical history needed, it appears that carbon is the most promising material yet for the tissue interface of transcutaneous devices. For this reason, carbon dental implants, carbon electrical connector seals for wiring to implanted electrodes for artificial hearing, seeing, and neurological devices, and carbon transcutaneous skeletal attachments to an external prosthesis are being carefully studied while undergoing clinical trials.

---

*Available commercially under the trade name Pyrolite Carbon—CarboMedics, Austin, Texas 78752.

A more recent development in the production of an isotropic carbon coating involves the use of a catalyst at close to ambient temperatures to promote the carbon deposition, thus allowing a variety of substrate materials, including polymers, to be coated. Referred to as ULTI carbon (ultra low temperature isotropic carbon),* it can be applied in a thin (<1.0 μm), tough, impermeable coating to impart improved thromboresistance to the fabrics of heart valve sewing rings and vascular prostheses or to invoke improved tissue response around metal implants.

Composites

The idea of using two or more materials as a composite, to obtain improved structural results, is quite old. The use of iron reinforcing rods in concrete is a man-made example. Nature's composition of bone is a remarkable composite: crystals of a calcium mineral—hydroxyapatite, $3Ca_3(PO_4)_2 \cdot Ca(OH)_2$—are held together with collagen, the same natural polymer making up tendons and skin, which acts in bone as a flexible glue. Consequently, although bone is hard, it is quite tough and has considerable resistance to bending or stretching.

Carbon-fiber-reinforced Carbon.   Carbon fiber/vitreous carbon composites may be fabricated by dipping carbon fiber into an ethanol solution of phenolic resin into which 20% by weight of micronized graphite has been suspended[14] after rapid drying in an oven at 80°C. The treated material is pressed to shape in a heated mold, whereupon the phenolic resin sets and the molded shape is removed from the mold.

The composite is then carbonized in an inert atmosphere by heating gradually to 1100°C or higher, thus yielding a carbon part which is about as convenient to produce, yet far tougher, than products made from the vitreous carbon material alone. Such parts will be useful for custom-made maxillofacial implants, particularly since molds can be cast from easily worked dental impressions or wax modeling materials.

Carbon-fiber-reinforced Ultra High Molecular Weight Polyethylene.
UHMW polyethylene has been described as having the best combination of properties to act as one of the articulating components of the

---

*Available commercially under the trade name Biolite Carbon—CarboMedics, Inc., Austin, Texas 78752.

metal-polymer interface of joint prostheses. However, as stable as UHMW polyethylene is, some degradation of the polymer takes place when it is implanted in the body, and when subjected to cyclic bending, gross fracture can occur.[15]

Significant reinforcement of the UHMW polyethylene may be achieved by the addition of carbon fibers to the molding compound. A special UHMW polyethylene, known as POLY TWO,* is reinforced with high strength carbon fibers having diameters ranging from 6 to 15 μm and averaging approximately 3 mm in length (Fig. 1-1). A proprietary molding procedure is used to achieve minimum thermal degradation of the polymer, minimum mechanical damage to the carbon fibers, and a good interfacial bond between the two so that

---

*Trademark, Zimmer, U.S.A., Warsaw, IN.

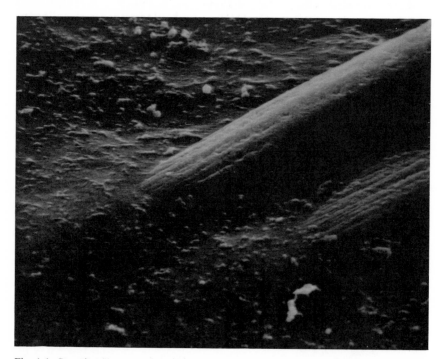

Fig. 1-1. Scanning electron microscope study of carbon fiber reinforcement and ultra high molecular weight polyethylene matrix interface ($\times$2500). The high strength fibers are 6–15 μm in diameter and approximately 3 mm long. They are randomly oriented. (*Courtesy of Zimmer, U.S.A.*)

maximum reinforcement results. Zimmer reports that a 15% carbon fiber loading improves compressive strength over 20%, flexural modulus close to 100%, wear by over 30%, and resistance to cold flow by more than 1000%. Biocompatibility of the POLY TWO composite is excellent.

Carbon Fiber–Polytetrafluoroethylene Composite. Proplast* is an ultraporous (70–90% by volume) implant material composed of Teflon and carbon fibers. It has the appearance and resiliency of a black felt sponge. It is easily carved to shape with a scalpel and can be safely sterilized by autoclaving. The carbon fibers present a highly wettable surface to body fluids; thus tissue growth, which serves to stabilize the implant, takes place rapidly. The wettable characteristic also allows Proplast to be bonded to metal or plastic prostheses in order to secure fixation to adjoining tissue. Proplast has found applications in maxillofacial, otologic, orthopedic, and plastic surgery.

A NATURAL POLYMER

Collagen is a generic term for the main supportive material of skin, tendon, cartilage, and connective tissue. It represents a group of fibrous proteins composed largely of three amino acids: glycine, proline, and hydroxyproline.

| Glycine | Proline | Hydroxyproline |

Collagen fibers are laid down by fibroblasts in the body in definite patterns, according to the requirements of the particular tissue (e.g., parallel in tendons, woven pattern in skin, etc.).

Collagen may be chemically cross-linked in order to stabilize it. This is what happens when hides are tanned to become leather. The collagen

*Trademark, Vitek, Inc., Houston, TX.

fibers of porcine heart valves are stabilized by using glutaraldehyde as the cross-linking agent. These natural valves have become quite popular as replacements for diseased human heart valves.

On the other hand, collagen may be made soluble by controlled proteolytic digestion.[16] The resulting, almost clear, viscous solution of collagen will spontaneously form a white opaque firm gel within ten minutes upon warming to 37° C. It has been used for the repair of soft tissue contour defects in humans;[17] upon injection into the site requiring augmentation, body heat quickly causes gelation with resultant preservation of contour reconstruction.

METALS

The use of metal implants goes back to ancient times. They were limited then to gold, silver, and copper which were easy metals to work but had insufficient strength for internal fixation purposes. In addition, copper had poor biocompatibility. It was not until the 1930s that advancing metallurgical technology and greatly improved surgical techniques began an era of expanding use of metal alloys in bone and joint replacement.

The successful long term performance of metal implants is dependent on a combination of properties which are difficult to achieve; along with the biocompatibility which all implant materials must exhibit, metals must blend toughness and strength with total corrosion resistance and, in the case of joints, outstanding wear resistance.

The principal metals used in joint prostheses today include titanium and its alloys, cobalt-chromium alloys, and stainless steel. Tantalum, gold, and platinum are used in smaller quantities for special applications.

Titanium

Titanium, especially the aluminum-vanadium alloy Ti-6Al-4V,* is rapidly becoming the structural implant metal of choice because of a very desirable combination of properties. In comparison with other structural implantable metals Ti-6Al-4V is the most biocompatible, the lightest, strongest, and the most corrosion[18] and fatigue resistant. Its

---

*Tivanium—trademark, Zimmer U.S.A., Warsaw, IN.

modulus of elasticity, the measure of the stiffness of a material, is roughly one-half of the others and therefore closer to bone (Table 1-1). This would lead to a more even application of a load stress at the implant-bone interface. Titanium is used in the replacement of joints and bone, and in fracture fixation devices. It is also used to encase and hermetically seal implantable energy packs such as the pulse generators of heart pacemakers. Heart valve components and some maxillofacial and dental implants are also made of titanium alloys.

Cobalt-Chromium Alloys

Cobalt-chromium alloys exhibit good wear and corrosion resistance as well as an acceptable level of biocompatibility. The original cast alloys lacked sufficient strength and fatigue resistance for rigorous applications such as the femoral stem of a hip prosthesis. More recent alloys which can be hot or cold worked have much improved properties and would be preferred over the titanium alloys when wear resistance is an important factor. These include Vitallium* a high cobalt-chromium alloy, Wrought T-Zimaloy (ASTM designation F-90) which is a cobalt-chromium-nickel-tungsten alloy (19–21% Cr, 9–11% Ni, 14–16% W), a multiphase alloy designated MP35N† (35% Co, 20% Cr, 35% Ni, 10% Mo), and a precipitation hardening wrought cobalt-nickel-chromium-titanium alloy[19] (40% Co, 18% Cr, 37% Ni, 5% Ti) which is claimed to be superior to other structural metal implants except for its resistance to crevice corrosion. In addition, cobalt-nickel-chromium-molybdenum-titanium alloy‡ (33–37% Ni, 19–21%, Cr, 9–10.5% Mo, .65–1% Ti) is claimed to have optimum mechanical and corrosion properties, proved by the history of over 100,000 implants between 1972 and 1976.[20]

Stainless Steel

316L, a low carbon austenitic stainless steel (17–20% Cr, 10–14% Ni, 2–4% Mo, 2% Mn), is the preferred stainless for prosthetic use. Although 316L stainless steel when coldworked is a strong, tough material, it is more susceptible to corrosion, particularly crevice

---

*Trademark, Howmedica, Inc., Rutherford, NJ.
†Standard Pressed Steel Company, U.S.A.
‡Protasul 10—Sulzer Brothers Limited, Switzerland.

corrosion, and to fatigue fracture than the titanium or the cobalt-chromium alloys. In addition to its use in skeletal repair, stainless steel has been used as the conductors in heart pacer and other electrical stimulator leads and also to encase the pulse generators.

Tantalum

Tantalum is an excellent material as far as its inertness and bio-compatibility is concerned. However, its application is limited because it is a very ductile metal of medium range strength properties. It has been used for the fashioning of plates to occlude openings in the skull, as well as for mesh in orbital floor repair and in some surgical staples.

Platinum

Platinum, because of its inertness and outstanding corrosion resistance, is the metal of choice for implantable electrodes. It is usually alloyed with 10% iridium as a hardening element.

CERAMICS

The inertness, excellent biocompatibility, and lack of corrosion of ceramic materials have led to their examination for use as endo-prostheses. Ceramics, such as alumina, are very strong in compression and extremely hard. However, their brittleness and their loss of strength when soaked in saline solution or implanted into the soft tissue of dogs or rabbits, as reported by Schmittgrund,[21] have led to a conservative approach to their application as implants.*

Interest in the use of ceramics has been strongest in Europe. Heinke[23] has reported on 600 ceramic-metal composite hip prostheses which have been implanted in Germany since 1974 with apparently satisfactory short term results. The acetabular components are made of Al_2O_3-ceramic, as are the femoral heads which are fixed to metal stems.

Bone tissue will not bond to Al_2O_3-ceramic; therefore, ceramic devices must be designed for mechanical anchoring. On the other hand, bone tissue will form a tight bond with bioglass material—however,

---

*Later work by Krainess and Knapp[22] related this to the effect of density of the ceramic. Densely sintered material prevented permeation of solution; consequently there was no loss of flexural strength. Material of only nominal density was permeable, and flexural strength dropped off greatly.

body fluids will eventually destroy the glass by dissolving it. There has been some interesting work done on the development of a glass-ceramic composite called Ceravital[24] which is stable yet will become anchored by attachment to bone tissue.

Silicon nitride, used in the production of high temperature turbine blades, is under observation as a bone and joint replacement material[25] in Sydney, Australia. It is stronger and less brittle than Al_2O_3-ceramic and can be machined easily into complex shapes.

A porous form of hydroxyapatite (occuring as coral) has been used as an implant material for the regeneration of bone.[26]

SAFETY TESTING OF IMPLANT MATERIALS

The determination of the safety of a prospective implant material is a knotty problem because it is impossible to duplicate exactly the total environment to which it will be subjected in the human body.

The physical properties of the candidate material may well suit the function of the device to which it is being applied. However, the absorption of lipids from body tissue, once the device has been implanted, and the action of various body enzymes and chemicals may promote degradation of the material leading to malfunction of the device and/or the production of by-products which would prove toxic to the host body.

A primary acute toxicity screening procedure for the toxicological evaluation of biomaterials, developed by the Materials Science Toxicology Laboratories (MSTL), University of Tennessee* and based on USPXIX† includes seven tests. The following three tests (condensed) are run directly on the material:

1. *Tissue Culture—Agar Overlay*: The object of this test is to detect the response of a mammalian monolayer cell culture to readily diffusible components from 1 cm^2 samples of material placed on the surface of the agar. Lysis or destruction of the cells is observed after incubation for 24 hours at 37° C. The area and extent of lysis is then noted and graded. This is a very sensitive test. It is also

---

*MSTL—John Autian, Ph.D., Director, University of Tennessee Medical Units, Memphis, TN 38163.
† United States Pharmacopeia XIX, "Biological Tests—Plastic Containers."

rapid and economical and therefore is considered ideal for preliminary screening. In all instances, MSTL reports, when a toxic response is recorded in the rabbit muscle implant, a cytotoxic response will be seen in the tissue culture procedure, whereas a cytotoxic response can be accompanied by a negative response in the rabbit muscle test because that test is not as sensitive.

2. *Rabbit Muscle Implant*: The test material is cut or formed roughly into a cylinder about 1½ cm long, fitting into a No. 15 trocar needle (about 1 mm in diameter). The needle is then introduced into a section of paravertebral muscle and withdrawn, leaving the material implanted in the muscle. After one week the animals are sacrificed and the sites of the implant are compared with a negative (polyethylene) and a positive (polyvinyl chloride containing 3% organotin stabilizer) control. The implant sites are then scored on the basis of tissue response from 0 (nonreactive) to 5 (marked reaction such as the positive control).

3. *Hemolysis—Rabbit Blood*: By using fresh, whole, oxalated, diluted rabbit blood with approximately 5 grams of material, if the percent hemolysis based on the average of three replicates if 5% or less, the material can be considered nonhemolytic.

The balance of the tests are run on extracts of the sample, using (a) saline, (b) polyethylene glycol 400, and (c) cottonseed oil. The extraction is conducted at 121°C for one hour in sealed tubes in an autoclave.

4. *Tissue Culture—Agar Overlay*: This is similar to the first test, except that 2 ml of extract are placed on the surface of sterile paper discs which have been previously laid on the agar. A negative control (solvent alone) is included on each plate, as well as a positive toxic control*; lysis is observed after incubation for 24 hours at 37°C. The area and extent of lysis are then noted and graded.

5. *Intracutaneous Injection in Rabbits*: This involves injection of .2 ml of extract intracutaneously at ten sites on the dorsal surface of

---

*A positive control is one containing a known toxic substance such as an organotin.

two rabbits, previously clipped of hair. The extract is injected on one side. On the other side, 20% ethyl alcohol is injected at five sites as a positive control; five additional sites are injected with the extracting medium alone. The sites of injection for the extract are scored as compared with controls at 24, 48, and 72 hours. The scoring system ranges from 0 (similar to the negative control) to 5 (equal to the positive control).

6. *Systemic Toxicity in Mice*: Injections of the extracts and the extracting medium are given, intravenously in the case of saline, intraperitoneally in the case of cottonseed oil and ethylene glycol 400. Five mice are injected with each substance. The dose level is 50 ml/kg. The response of mice injected with extract is compared to that of mice injected with extracting medium over a period of one week. This is the least sensitive of the series; consequently, any material producing a severe toxic response or death would be undesirable as in implant material.

7. *Tissue Culture—Inhibition of Cell Growth Assay*: Nine different sample weights per 20 ml of distilled water are extracted for one hour at 121° C in sealed tubes in an autoclave. Equal quantities of the extracts and double strength Eagle's medium are mixed, and 2 ml of each mixture are added to ten assay tubes containing a suspension of mouse fibroblast cells (strain L-929) having a cell density of 10^6 cells/ml. One-half of the tubes are incubated for 72 hours, centrifuged, and decanted; the other half are centrifuged and decanted immediately. There is a linear relationship between cell number and protein concentration. By using the colormetric method of Lowry[27] to determine the average protein content of each set of five tubes, the percent inhibition of cell growth may be obtained.

The biological response to each test is given a weighted value. The total of all responses is referred to as the cumulative toxicity response (CTI), the highest values for which is 1500. Naturally, the lowest possible toxicity values are the most desirable. A CTI of 100 or less is considered to have a low potential toxicity. Table 1-2 lists the lowest CTI values reported by MSTL on some of the commonly used biomaterials.

After primary acute toxicity screening, long term tests are normally

Table 1.2. Cumulative Toxicity Index (CTI) for Selected
Polymer Materials.

MATERIAL	CTI
Polymethyl methacrylate	30
Polycarbonate membrane	30
Epoxy	32
Polyurethane	40
Ethyl cellulose	56
Polysulfone	56
Polyethylene	65
Silicone rubber	81
Polyvinyl chloride (prepared with toxic agents)	763

run on dogs or larger animals, duplicating as closely as possible the procedure and device configuration to be used in humans. The length of such tests will depend on a number of factors, including the expected useful life of the device and the requirements of the FDA Bureau of Medical Devices and Diagnostic Products (BuDD). During the long term tests, biofunctionability, the ability of the device to perform in the bioenvironment in which it will be used, is continuously checked. Clinical trials on humans complete the series. It is not uncommon that design changes are found necessary during this stage of testing. The toxicological screening of materials for a new critical device and the biotesting of the device constitute at best time consuming, expensive procedures.

Upon approval by BuDD to market the new device, its manufacture must be carried out under conditions which will insure strict adherence to specifications, no contamination of materials, and complete traceability of each lot.

REFERENCES

1. Williams, D. F., and Roaf, R. *Implants in Surgery.* W. B. Saunders 1973, p. 257.
2. Kusy, R. P. Characterization of self-curing acrylic bone cements. *J. Biomed. Mat. Res.* **12**(3). 273 (1978).
3. Moyer, Robin: Blood without donors, Science 81, 16–17, June 81.
4. Spector, M., et al. A high-modulus polymer for porous orthopedic implants. *J. Biomed. Mat. Res.* **12**(5):665–677 (1978).
5. Rowe, V. K., Spencer, H. S., and Bass, S. L. Toxocological studies on certain commerical silicones. II. Two year dietary feeding of DC Antifoam A to rats. *Arch. Ind. Hyg. Occupational Med.* **1** :529–554 (1950).

6. Child, G. P., Paquin, H. O., and Deichman, W. B. Chronic toxicity of the methylpolysiloxane, DC Antifoam A in dogs. *Arch. Ind. Hyg. Occupational Med.* 3:479–482 (1951).
7. Paul, J., and Pover, W. F. R. The failure of absorption of DC Silcone Fluid 703 from the gastrointestinal tract of rats. *Brit. J. Ind. Med.* 17:149–154 (1960).
8. Hobbs, E. J., Keplinger, M. L., and Calandra, J. C. Toxicity of polydimethyl silixanes in certain environmental systems. *Envir. Res.* 10:397–406 (1975).
9. Lynch, W. *Handbook of Silicone Rubber Fabrication.* New York: Van Nostrand Reinhold, 1978.
10. Jenkins, G. M., and Kawamura, K., *Polymeric Carbons—Carbon Fibre, Glass and Char.* Cambridge University Press, 1976.
11. Jenkins, D. H. R. The repair of tendons with carbon fiber. *International Bomaterials Symposium*, Philadelphia, April 1976.
12. Bokros, J. C., et al. Prostheses made of carbon. *Chemical Technology* 7:40–49 (1977).
13. Meffert, R. M. Periodontal aspects of implants. *Oral Implant* 6(4):558 (1977).
14. Jenkins, G. M., and Grigson, C. J. The fabrication of artifacts out of glassy carbon and carbon-fiber-reinforced carbon for biomedical applications. *J. Biomed. Mat. Res.* 13(3):372–394 (1979).
15. Weightman, B., et al. The fracture of UHMWP in the human body. *J. Biomed. Mat. Res.* 13:669–672 (1979).
16. Stenzel, K. H., Miyata, T., and Rubin, A. L. Collagen as a biomaterial. *Ann. Rev. Biophys. Bioeng.* 3:231 (1974).
17. Knapp, T. R., Luck, E., and Daniels, J. R., Behavior of solubolized collagen as a bioimplant. *J. Surg. Res.* 23:96–105 (1977).
18. Thompson, N. G., Buchanan, R. A., and Lemons, J. E. In vitro corrosion of Ti-6 Al-4V and type 316L stainless steel when galvanically coupled with carbon. *J. Biomed. Mat. Res.* 13(1):35–44 (1979).
19. Cahoon, J. R., and Hill, L. D. Evaluation of a precipitation hardened wrought cobalt-nickel-chromium-titanium alloy for surgical implants. *J. Biomed. Mat. Res.* 12(6):805–821 (1978).
20. Süry, P., and Semlitsch, M. Corrosion behaviour of cast and forged cobalt based alloys for double-alloy joint endoprotheses. *International Biomaterials Symposium*, New Orleans, April 1977.
21. Schmittgrund, G. D., et al. In vivo and in vitro changes in strength of orthopaedic calcium aluminates. *J. Biomed. Mat.* Res. (4):437 (1973).
22. Krainess, F. E., and Knapp, W. J. Strength of a dense alumina ceramic after aging in vitro. *J. Biomed. Mat. Res.* 12:241–246 (1978).
23. Heinke, G., et al; Direct Anchorage of Al_2O_3-ceramic hip components: three years of clinical experience and results of further animal studies. *J. Biomed. Mat. Res.* 12:57–65 (1978).
24. Blencke, B. A., et al; Compatibility and long-term stability of glass-ceramic implants. *J. Biomed. Mat. Res.* 12:307–316 (1978).
25. *Chemical Week*, p. 69, Sept. 26, 1979.
26. Holmes, R. E. Bone regeneration within a coralline hydroxyapatite implant. *Plastic and Reconstructive Surgery* 626–633 (1979).
27. Lowry, O. H., et al. Protein measurement with the folin phenol reagent. *J. Biol. Chem.* 193:265 (1951).

2
SKELETON AND JOINT PROSTHESES

The animal skeleton plays three important roles: it protects vital organs such as the brain, eyes, and viscera; it maintains the shape of the body; but most important, it translates muscular exertion into a great variety of movements—some of them quite complicated and subtle.

In order to function most effectively, nature has evolved in skeletal bone a composite material which combines great strength, toughness, and resilience with light weight. Bone is composed mainly of minute crystals of a calcium mineral (hydroxyapatite) firmly bonded with collagen fiber. Collagen is also the material of cartilage and tendon; when boiled out of old bones, it becomes the animal glue still used in the furniture and packaging industries, although to a great extent it has been replaced by synthetic adhesives. So, in effect, in bone we have a material composed of many rigid particles bonded with an elastic glue and thus exhibiting superior shock resistance.

Microscopic examination of bone shows it to be quite porous in structure even in its most dense condition. The porous structure of bone not only contributes to its low weight to strength ratio but makes it more resistant to stress crack growth (see Fig. 2-1). A long bone such as the femur (thigh bone, Fig. 2-2), which is the largest bone in the body and is subjected in the active human to great stress, is tubular in construction. An outer hard layer is referred to as compact tissue; an inner, more spongy layer is called cancellous tissue. Marrow which contains erythroblasts, from which red corpuscles of the blood are derived, fills the cavity of the bone and also occupies the spaces of the cancellous tissue. Numerous blood vessels traverse minute orifices in the bone. Nerves and some lymphatic vessels also accompany the arteries into its interior.

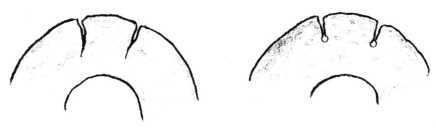

Fig. 2-1. It is well known that crack growth in a material can be stopped by drilling a hole at the leading edge of a crack. Cancellous tissue of the bone combats crack growth in the same manner, thus increasing its toughness.

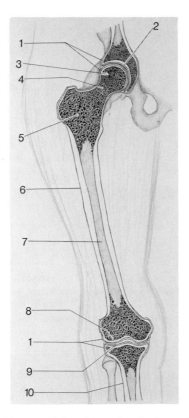

Fig. 2-2. Structure of a long bone and joints, illustrating the femur, hip, and knee joints: (1) articular capsule lined with synovial membrane which produces the synovial fluid for joint lubrication; (2) articular cartilage; (3) head of femur; (4) neck of femur; (5) cancellous or spongy bone; (6) shaft of femur, compact bone; (7) medullary canal; (8) femoral condyles (two); (9) articular surfaces of tibia; two concave tuberosities, (the semilunar cartilages surround the articular surfaces serving to deepen them); (10) tibia.

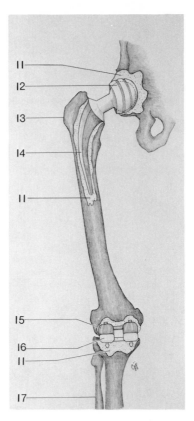

Fig. 2-3 The femur; illustrating total hip implant and surface replacement type of knee implant: (11) acrylic bone cement; (12) ultra high molecular weight polyethylene acetabular cup; (13) great trochanter; (14) metal femoral component; (15) metal runners of femoral knee component; (16) UHMW polyethylene tibial platforms; (17) fibula.

JOINTS

There are a variety of articulating joints in the body. These include the simple hinge type found in the fingers which allows approximately a 90° bend in one direction only. The saddle joint of the spinal vertebra allows a slight rocking motion from side to side and front to back along with some rotation, the multiple effect of many vertebrae leading to a high degree of flexibility. The ball and socket joint found in the hip allows a great freedom of movement as well as the ability to function under a heavy load. Furthermore, the elbow exhibits a combination of hinge action with rotation.

The articulating surface of the joint is covered with a layer of cartilage which has a microporous structure, although it is smooth and glossy in appearance. Articulating joints are entirely surrounded by a tough synovial membrane which secretes a transparent viscid fluid having the consistency of the white of an egg and known as synovial fluid. The synovial fluid fills the joint spaces and is absorbed by the microporous cartilage layer.

During the sliding, rolling action of the joint, the pressure points on the cartilaginous surface are continually changing position. At the point of pressure, synovial fluid weeps out of the microporous structure of the cartilage to form a fluid lubricating layer. As the pressure point changes position, synovial fluid is reabsorbed to be ready for the next cycle. Bioengineers have a long way to go to match such an effective system. Coefficients of friction as low as .005 have been claimed for some human joints.

Etiology Leading to Joint Replacement

Arthritis is one of man's most common and least understood diseases. There is no known cure, and only palliative relief is available in some cases through the use of anti-inflammatory drugs or electronic neurostimulation (chapter 8). When a person is suffering severe arthritic pain or deformity, or has little range of movement, the use of an artificial joint is indicated. The use of a joint prosthesis avoids the sometimes harmful side effects of high doses of steroids and other palliative drugs. Joint prostheses are also indicated after fracture, when difficulty in healing is encountered.

Total Hip Replacement

The work of John Charnley, F.R.S.C., during the 1950s in England led to the development of the first practical, artificial hip joint. Many modifications of this device are available today. One is the Müller type illustrated in Fig. 2–4. This design features an acetabular cup molded of ultra high molecular weight polyethylene* and a metal femoral component having a spherical head which articulates within the cup. The articulating surfaces of the two components must be mirror

---

*Molecular weight = 6–8×10^6.

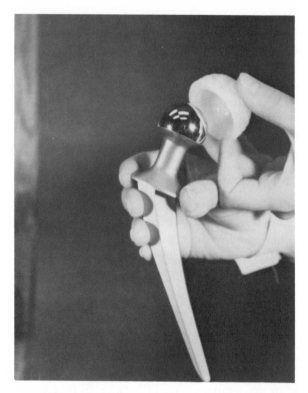

Fig. 2–4. Zimmer total hip prosthesis. The acetabular cup molded of UHMW polyethylene has a microfinish of 20 millionths of an inch on the articulating surface to provide the lowest possible coefficient of friction and a long service life. The outer surface of the cup is undercut to provide mechanical attachment by bone cement. Radiographic wires are molded in place.

finished to reduce friction and wear to a minimum. The combination of polyethylene with metal results in a much lower coefficient of friction and less wear than metal on metal.

More recently, a composite of UHMW polyethylene reinforced with pyrolitic carbon fibers has been used for the acetabular cup. A significant improvement in compressive strength, wear properties, creep, and resistance to fatigue is realized over the plain UHMW polyethylene. Femoral components are often made of stainless steel or chromium-cobalt alloys; however, there is a trend toward the use of titanium alloys because they exhibit the best known combination of toughness, light weight, corrosion resistance, and biocampatibility of any metal.

Acrylic Bone Cement

The results of total hip arthroplasty have been quite beneficial to people who have, for all practical purposes, lost the function of their natural joint. It is estimated that at least 100,000 hip replacements are performed annually in in the United States. As reliable as the current procedure is, there are a number of shortcomings which call for improvement. The foremost of these is the method of attachment to the bone. The standard method is by the use of an acrylic bone cement. This is similar to the acrylic impression material used by dentists. There is no actual adhesion of the bone cement to the bone tissue; the attachment is strictly mechanical. It holds because of interdigitation with the porous structure of the cancellous bone. There are several factors which may contribute to the loosening.

The primary factor is the composition and characteristics of the bone cement itself. The cement is supplied as a two-component system. One package contains methyl methacrylate polymer in powder form, together with a small amount of cross-linking agent, also a powder. The other package contains methyl methacrylate monomer, a fluid. When the contents of the two packages are mixed, a doughy consistency is obtained for the first several minutes. While doughy, the bone cement is forced into the cavity, and the implant is positioned and held in place. Polymerization of the methyl methacrylate monomer proceeds rapidly and the cement becomes rigid. The polymerization reaction is exothermic and is accompanied by a considerable liberation of heat. Polymerization temperatures of over 100°C have been reported, which is high enough to cause necrosis of the immediately adjacent bone tissue. Accompanying polymerization and the ensuing cooling is a volumetric shrinkage of about 4%. Between the necrosis and the shrinkage, there is the early possiblity of loosening at the prosthesis-bone interface. The initial loosening may not be of consequence, but the continued abrasion of the two mating surfaces can produce particulate debris which would speed the abrading and necrosis, thus contributing to progressive loosening of the joint. Another drawback of the acrylic cement mixture is that the monomer is highly toxic. Although most of the monomer becomes polymerized, some is always available on the surface of the final product. Apart from some serious consequences of getting minute amounts into the blood stream, which at worst could cause cardiac arrest, the monomer may cause necrosis in adjacent bone tissue which, as has been discussed, can be the precursor of loosening. In normal use, the force on the hip can run as much as four times the weight of the person; consequently, an unattended loose prosthesis could eventually cause splitting of the bone.

An approach which has been suggested by Rijke et al.[1] is the mixing of a crystalline material into the acrylic cement. The crystalline material such as sugar should be insoluble in the cement but readily absorbed by the body. Upon absorption it leaves a porous layer of cement into which bone tissue growth can take place, thus improving the bond. Also since the total amount of acrylic cement is reduced, the effects of both exothermic heat and monomer would be reduced in proportion to the amount of added crystalline material. Although there would be some loss of strength, presumably this would be outweighed by the other advantages.

Another approach for prosthesis fixation has been tried, reportedly with a good degree of success, by a French orthopedic surgeon, Gerald A. Lord. The stem of the femoral component is surfaced with a coral-like texture of tiny balls machined from a cobalt-chromium alloy (see Fig. 2-5). Trabecular bone forms and affixes to the irregular surface. Lord reports success in several hundred cases in over five years. An osteogenic process definitely occurs at the bone-prosthesis interface to give firm attachment. The drawback to this method is that the surgical technique must be very precise and the patient must be kept immobile until the new bone growth has formed and firmly fixed the prosthesis. This may amount to several weeks.

A certain degree of success in animal studies has been achieved through the use of porous metals,[2,3] porous ceramics, and porous UHMW polyethylene. Pore sizes to encourage bone ingrowth should be 100 μm or greater, and dead space between the porous implant surface and the cut surface of the bone should be no greater than 1–2 mm.[4] Although ceramics have excellent bioacceptability and superior inertness, the friability of a porous type would be a drawback.

Polyethylene, on the other hand, could combine a desirable combination of inertness and toughness, and has seen some successful clinical applications.[5] A unique method of attachment of a dense ceramic device may be seen in Fig. 2-6. The use of ceramics for implants has been pursued more extensively in Europe than in North

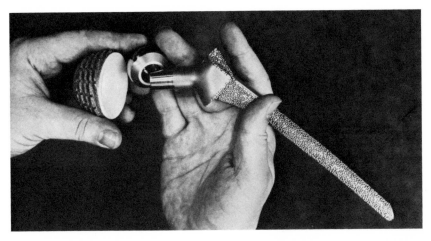

Fig. 2-5 Total hip prosthesis introduced at the APAS hospital in France in which the stem, of the femoral component has a rough surface consisting of a multitude of tiny cast-on balls. The acetabular cup has a rough outer metal surface with a highly polished polyethylene inner lining. For older patients the femoral component is one piece, but for young patients the head (as illustrated) is removable: if the ball or cup needs changing, the stem does not have to be removed. *Photo*: (*Courtesy of the American Academy of Orthopedic Surgeons, Chicago, IL.*) Text reprinted from *Medical World News* Copyright © 1978 McGraw-Hill, Inc.

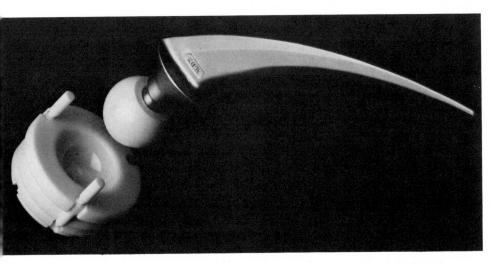

Fig. 2-6. A ceramic metal composite total hip prosthesis. (*Courtesy of Mark Lindenhof*)

America. The acetabular cup is made of dense, high purity Al_2O_3-ceramic* and is intended for direct, cement free fixation[7]. The pins crossing the undercuts are used for initial stabilization of the component during bone remodeling. The ball of the femur component is of the same material and is fixed to the metal stem by a self-locking cone. The metal stem is anchored in the femur in the conventional manner using bone cement.

A cover of polyester mesh is used on some small implants such as finger joints to promote the ingrowth of anchoring fibrous tissue.

Until more dependable methods of attachment are developed and the life span of an artificial hip can be safely predicted to be over ten years, young active patients who would quickly outlast their prosthesis should not be considered candidates except as a last resort. The possiblity of using transplanted cadaver allografts of bone and cartilage to reconstruct damaged sections of joints as an alternative for young people has been reported recently in the medical press.[6]

Total Knee Replacement

The action of the natural knee is more complex than the hip and is difficult to reproduce in a prosthesis. Besides its apparent hinge action, which allows flexion and extension, the knee structure allows a polycentric rotation which helps diminish the normal torque of the leg while walking.

The available knee prostheses can be classified broadly into two categories: a surface replacement type and a stabilizing type. An example of the former (illustrated in Fig. 2-3) is shown in Fig. 2-7. Existing ligaments are left intact; only the load bearing surfaces are replaced. The femoral condyles are replaced by two metal alloy runners which fit into and slide in polyethylene tibial platforms single units may be used if only one of the weight bearing surfaces is eroded). In this way some of the polycentric motion of the knee is preserved.

The loss of mobility of the knee joint is a severe deterrent to the function of the leg. When the joint is severely damaged and chronic pain is experienced, the stabilizing type of joint shown in Fig. 2-8 is used. This hinged type of knee joint requires a radical surgical

---

*FRIALIT—registered trademark, Friedrichsfeld GmbH., Steinzeng und Kunstoffwerke, Medizinal-Technik, Mannheim, West Germany.

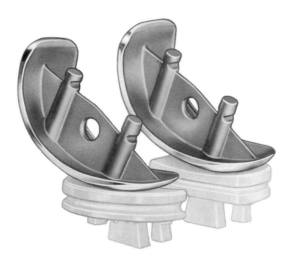

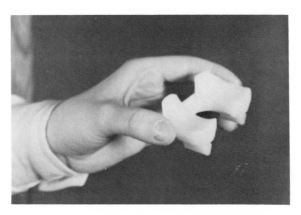

Fig. 2–7. Zimmer knee implants for replacement of the articulation surfaces. The metal alloy runners are shown (*top*) along with the UHMW polyethylene tibial platform (*bottom*). (*Courtesy of Zimmer, U.S.A.*)

approach in which the cruciate ligaments, femoral condyles, and tibial platform are removed, and the bone is resected. Both types of knee replacement (Figs. 2–7 and 2–8) are currently being fixed with acrylic cement.

None of the currently used devices replaces the patella. Although thousands of total knee replacements have been made, the general

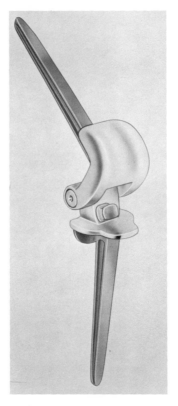

Fig. 2-8. Zimmer Offset Hinge total knee implant. (*Courtesy of Zimmer, U.S.A.*)

opinion in the orthopedic field is that this step should be taken as a last resort. Although pain is relieved and motion restored, a person cannot run, squat, or kneel. Also, the knee is more prone to infection than the hip.

Total Elbow Replacement

The elbow (Fig. 2-9) is an even more difficult joint than the knee as far as duplicating the complex combination of motion which includes flexion, extension, angular displacement, and rotation of the ulna upon the humerus. Loss of use of the elbow will severely reduce hand function and the ability to perform an almost infinite number of intricate tasks. As a result of its importance there are about a dozen different elbow prostheses on the market. Most of these are hinge type

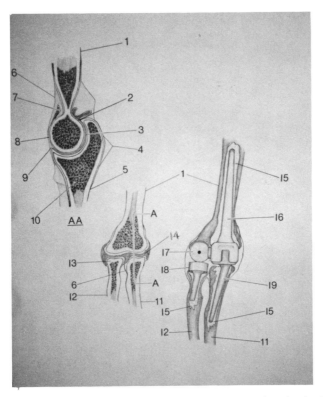

Fig. 2-9. *left*: Structure of the elbow; *right*: diagrammatic representation of an implanted AMC Radio-capitellar total elbow prosthesis (Volz). (1) Humerus, (2) trochlea, (3) ulnar semilunar notch, (4) olecranon, (5) ulna, (6) synovial membrane, (7) synovial fluid, (8) articular cartilage, (9) compact bone, (10) cancellous tissue, (11) ulna, (12) radius, (13) capitulum of the radius, (14) articular cavity, (15) bone cement, (16) humeral stem component, (17) metal alloy capitellar sphere—an integral part of the humeral component, (18) radial head component fabricated from high density polyethylene, (19) ulnar stem component.

prostheses, such as the Coonrad total elbow (Fig. 2–10), which replace the ulnar-humeral joint. Although they have been effective in relieving intractable pain and offer increased range of motion and stability, they cannot be used in the performance of heavy work or athletics because of the risk of loosening the cement-bone bond.

A new total elbow in which both radial-humeral and ulnar-humeral sections of the joint are replaced is a development of Robert G. Volz, orthopedic surgeon at the College of Medicine, University of Arizona. The Volz design, shown in Fig. 2–9, allows pronation and supination

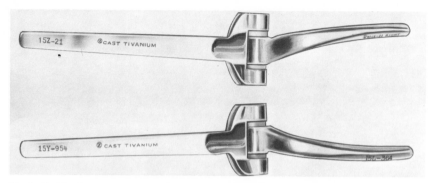

Fig. 2–10. The Coonrad elbow, developed by Dr. Ralph W. Coonrad of Duke University in 1970, was the first to use high density polyethylene interposed between the metal hinge parts. It is a rigid hinge type and is generally implanted when there is actual bone loss. (*Courtesy of Zimmer, U.S.A.*)

of the forearm in a near normal manner. It is intended to permit three planes of motion at the humeral-ulnar articulation. At the same time, the soft tissue envelope is preserved for its utilization in the dissipation of stresses at the joint interface. Because the lifting of a weight puts much more stress on the elbow than on the hand, the inclusion of a radial head component, which can act as a buttress to preventing angular distortion of the forearm upon the arm, reduces these high stresses by approximately half. The patient is then equipped with a reasonably naturally functioning elbow, which has a higher safety factor as far as loosening in use is concerned.

Total Wrist

Silicone rubber or pyrolite carbon coated implants are used to replace separate articulation surfaces of the wrist such as the distal radial head, distal ulnar head, and the semilunar and scaphoid bones (see Fig. 2–11). The major problem, until recently, with total wrist arthroplasty, has been the determination of the optimal location for the axes of motion of the implant so that they would coincide closely with the normal site of the axes of motion of the wrist. A wrist prosthesis, developed by Dr. Robert S. Hamas[8] and designed to eliminate this problem, is shown in Fig. 2–12. The axes of motion of the prosthesis (Fig. 2–12a) are offset from the axes of the anchoring stems. When the anchoring stems are centered in the medullary canals of the third

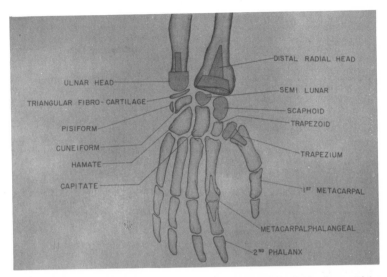

Fig. 2-11. Palmar view of left hand and wrist showing location of silastic* implants which replace the articular surfaces. There is no positive attachment to the interfacing bone. They can be replaced easily if required.

metacarpal and the distal radius (Fig. 2-12b), the axes of motion are at the optimal location for any size of wrist. Since the offsets are in different directions for right and left wrists, it is necessary to have both right and left devices. This "precentered" total wrist prosthesis greatly simplifies the operative procedure and seems to lead to excellent results.

Use of Rubber in Joint Replacement

Arthritic deformities of the fingers are fairly common. In addition to the usual pain and loss of function, they are often quite unsightly. Finger prostheses made from silicone rubber have been successfully used to replace proximal interphalangeal (PIP) and metacarpophalangeal (MP) joints (Fig. 2-11). One type is a one-piece, flexible design with intramedullary stems. There is no attempt to gain attachment to the bone; it is claimed that the sliding action or pistoning in the intramedullary cavity gives a more natural finger action and allows easy replacement when necessary.[9] Another type has an open

---

*Silastic—registered trademark, Dow Corning Corp., Midland, Mich.

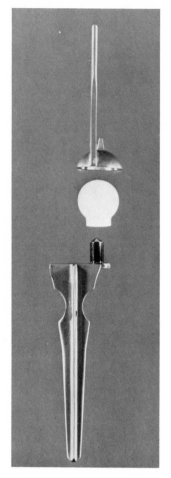
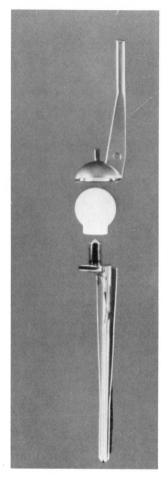

(a)

Fig. 2–12. "Precentered" total wrist prosthesis (Hamas).

mesh Dacron fabric attached to the intramedullary stems to encourage tissue ingrowth with resultant anchoring to the bone.[10] An example of the latter is illustrated in Fig. 2–13. Application of this style of implant in the restoration of a hand disfigured by arthritis is pictured in Fig. 2–14.

There have been flex failures of both of these types of silicone rubber prostheses. There is promising new polyolefin elastomer which is biocompatible and demonstrates an extraordinary flex life. Clinical trials are presently being run on Lord finger joints containing this material (Fig. 2–15).

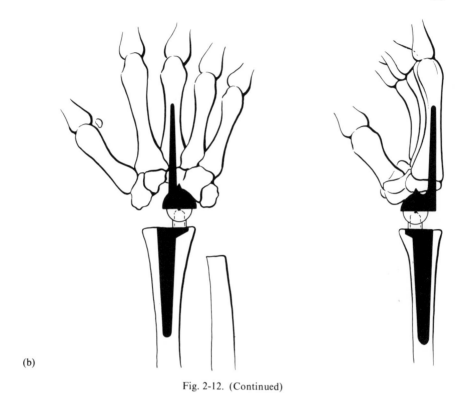

(b)

Fig. 2-12. (Continued)

Using the basic technology it developed for elastomeric helicopter rotor bearings, the Lord Corporation designed this finger joint prosthesis. It consists of titanium alloy stems sized to fit the medullary cavity of the phalange or metacarpal. Connecting the stems is the polyolefin elastomer which is bonded to the stems and to the rigid central piece. The purpose of the insert is to provide normal finger kinematics, to increase the axial load carrying capability, to increase the lateral and shear stiffnesses, and to provide for a more even strain distribution in the elastomer. If the clinical results prove to be as good as animal trials have indicated, we should expect to find polyolefin elastomers applied in combination with rigid materials toward improvement of other artificial joints as well.

Total shoulder replacement presents a challenging design problem. While the joint is a ball and socket type, it is unlike the stable, deeply socketed hip joint. The glenoid cavity provides only a shallow depression for the large spherical head of the humerus in order to allow

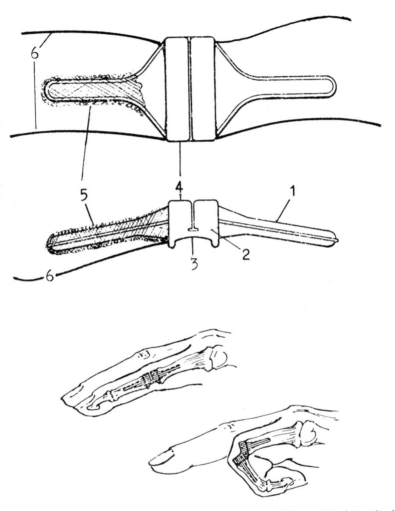

Fig. 2-13. Design features of Niebauer finger joint: (1) molded silicone rubber integral unit; (2) polyester reinforcement molded in place; (3) thin hinge section for easy flexing and long flex life; (4) buttress to prevent buckling of hinge when finger is in extension; (5) both stems are covered with polyester fabric to gain attachment to the bone through the invasion of fibrous tissue; (6) integral suture ties provide immediate fixation when tied through small drill holes in the metacarpal and phalangial bones. The sketch to the right shows the position of the prosthesis with the finger extended and with it flexed. Artificial finger joints come in various sizes. (*From Handbook of Silicone Rubber Fabrication, New York: Van Nostrand Reinhold,* 1978).

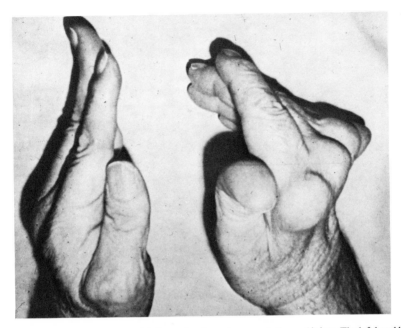

Fig. 2-14. An arthritic right hand deformed at the metacarpophalangeal joints. The left hand has been restored to normal appearance and near normal function by removal of this diseased joints and their replacement with Niebauer rubber finger joint prostheses. (*Courtesy J. Leonard Goldner, M.D. Duke University Medical Center, and Sutter Biomedical,Inc.*) San Diego, Ca.

the widest range of movement of all the joints. The shoulder joint is capable of movement of every type—forward, backward, abduction, adduction, circumduction, and rotation. The numerous rotator ligaments of the shoulder act as a tendinous socket which grasps the globular humeral head, allowing its articulation without dislocation. It is not surprising that this sacrifice of bony stability at the shoulder, combined with the requirement of great mobility, has led to the limited success of shoulder implants.

A shoulder prosthesis described as a "floating-socket" system[11] has given some promising results in limited clinical testing. A non-dislocatable, dual spherical bearing system, consisting of a small sphere within a larger sphere with their centers offset to provide a floating fulcrum, allows a range of motion in excess of anatomical limits. Consequently, the motion is limited by soft tissue structures rather than by mechanical impingement which would stress and

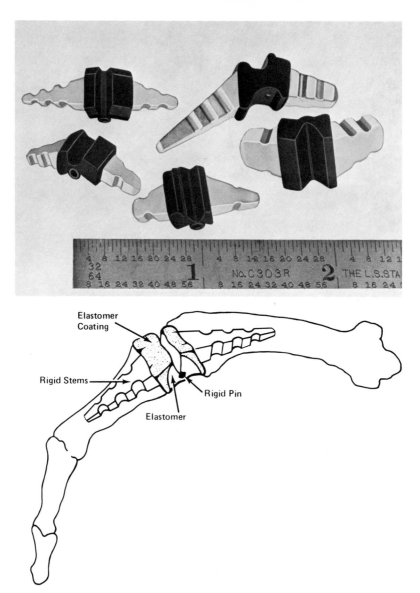

Fig. 2–15. *Lord Finger Joint.* Using the basic technology it developed for elastomeric helicopter rotor bearings, the Lord Corporation designed a finger joint prosthesis. It consists of titanium alloy stems sized to fit the medullary cavity of the phalange or metacarpal. Connecting the stems is the polyolefin elastomer which is bonded to the stems and to the rigid central piece. The purpose of the insert is to provide normal finger kinematics, to increase the axial load-carrying capability, to increase the lateral and shear stiffnesses, and to provide for a more even strain distribution in the elastomer.

ultimately loosen the attachment. The device is constructed of metal alloy and high density polyethylene; there is no metal to metal contact.

A total ankle prosthesis has a talar component of metal alloy which articulates with an UHMW polyethylene distal tibial component.

Modifications of the silicone rubber prostheses used for replacement of the joints of the hand are available for use in the foot[12,13] (Fig. 2–16).

The successful use of silicone and polyolefin elastomers for the fabrication of finger joints may very well be the forerunner of the application of elastomers in the design of other artificial joints. The energy damping characteristics and the ability to distribute strain more evenly than rigid materials will certainly contribute to a more rugged, longer service life.

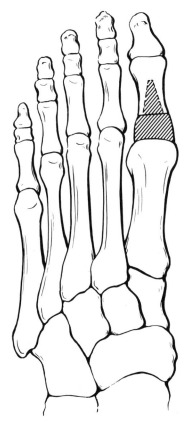

Fig. 2–16. The Silastic Great Toe Implant from Dow Corning Corporation is designed for use following surgery for bunions.

IMPLANT FOR ORTHOTICS

Direct Attachment of an External Prothesis of the Skeletal System

An age-old problem for the lower limb amputee has been to obtain a satisfactory external prosthesis. Despite new resilient materials which allow the molding of the prothesis socket to the shape of the leg stump, the wearing of an artificial leg can be rather uncomfortable to say the least. Research with the biocarbon materials discussed elsewhere in this book has shown that they have long term promise as effective transcutaneous materials. With the potential of a viable transcutaneous seal available, the Rehabilitation Engineering Center at Ranchos Los Amigos Hospital in Downey, California has collaborated with the Kennedy Space Center in developing a satisfactory method of attaching a prosthesis to the skeleton (Fig. 2–17). The metal alloy tibial component* was fixed in the intermedullary canal with methyl methacrylate bone cement. The LTI carbon transcutaneous section was bonded to the tibial component† which contains a latching device for attaching the prosthesis. This device has been implanted in the leg of an amputee.[14,15]

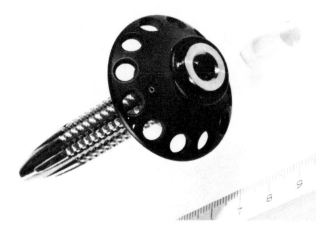

Fig. 2–17. Transcutaneous skeletal prosthesis attachment. The metal alloy tibial component* was fixed in the intermedullary canal with methyl methacrylate bone cement. The LTI carbon transcutaneous section was bonded to the tibial component† which contains a latching device for attaching the prosthesis.

---

*Fabricated by Kennedy Space Center, NASA.
†By CarboMedics, Inc.

Tendon Prostheses

Successful tendon repair and reconstruction have been achieved through the use of silicone rubber tendon underlays and pulleys.[16] The implanted silicone prevents the adhesions which are often the plague of tendon surgery. Repair has been achieved by the use of full-length suture material encased in a Dacron-fabric-reinforced silicone rubber sheath having Dacron mesh and tabs for attachment.

Experiments on animals have demonstrated that pure carbon in a flexible, filamentous form of great tensile strength can be used successfully to induce the formation of new tendons.[17] When the tendon is replaced with filamentous carbon, the carbon fibers take over the tendon function for the first few weeks. During this period fibrous connective tissue is laid down alongside the carbon, and in approximately eight weeks a newly induced tendon takes over the action of the implant—the carbon implant has in fact played the part of a temporary scaffold or stent. Materials other than carbon do not appear to have this capability.

Muscle Implant

Skeletal muscles occur as pairs opposed to one another. They are capable only of producing tensile forces. It has been shown that experiments on animals that one muscle of an antagonistic pair can be replaced with a passive elastic implant and the pair can function in a practical manner.[18] The artificial muscle was fabricated from a crimped, stretchable Dacron inner tube, covered with a silicone rubber outer tube. The Dacron extended past the silicone on each end to form an attachment to the tendon.

Electrical Stimulation of Bone Growth

Electrical stimulation of bone growth has been used clinically for some time in the healing of complicated fractures which do not respond to standard treatment. Nonhealing fractures usually occur among the elderly or in young people with an inherited condition called pseudo-arthrosis of the tibia in which nerve defects block the healing. Without successful knitting of the break, the broken limb may eventually have to be amputated.

Investigators have long known that deformation of bone produces low voltage electrical currents, and in the 1950s Yasudo and Fukada demonstrated that electrical current stimulates bone formation. This principle has been successfully applied by Dr. Carl T. Brighton of the University of Pennsylvania to hundreds of patients who had poorly mending fractures, by inserting electrodes around the break, applying a plaster cast to the broken limb, and connecting the electrodes to a battery powered energy source which delivers a steady 10–20 μA of electricity. In about three months the electrodes are removed, and in another three months the limb is completely restored to full activity. Other early pioneers in the invasive application of electrical stimulation for bone growth are Dr. Robert O. Becker at Syracuse New York V.A. Hospital and Dr. Leroy S. Lavine at the State University of New York Downstate Medical Center

Dr. Andrew Bassett, chief of the orthopedic research labs at Columbia Presbyterian Medical Center, has taken a different tack. He has successfully applied electrial stimulation in a noninvasive manner to obtain solid bone growth. Bassett's method consists of placing two pads containing electrical coils, one on each side of the cast, and applying a pulsating current for 12 hours each day. Besides eliminating the surgery, Bassett reports a high success rate of about 80 percent in hundreds of cases.

It is conceivable that one of the main drawbacks of retention of orthopedic implants (the length of time for attachment by natural bone tissue ingrowth) will be overcome by speeding up the process through electrical stimulation.

REFERENCES

1. Rijke, A.M., et al. Porous acrylic cement. *J. Biomed. Mat. Res.* **11**:373–394 (1977).
2. Mooz, A., et al. Mechanical characteristics of the porous surface coated surgical implant alloy, Ti-6 Al-4V. *28th Can. Metal Physics Conf.* June, 1978.
3. Medley, J., et al. Development of a more compatible implant for hip hemiarthroplasty. *Trans. Fourth Ann. Meeting of the Society for Biomaterials*, San Antonio, Texas, April, 1978.
4. Swanson, S.A.V., and Freeman, M.A.R. *The Scientific Basis of Joint Replacement.* New York: Wiley, 1977.
5. Sauer, B.W. Stabilization of surgical implants with porous high density polyethylene. *National Tech Conference S.P.E.*, Denver, November 1977.
6. *Medical World News* 53 (1978).

7. Heinke, G. Direct anchorage of Al$_2$O$_3$-ceramic hip components: three years of clinical experience and results of further animal studies. *J. Biomed. Mat. Res.* **12**:57–65 (1978).
8. Hamas, R.S. A quantitative approach to total wrist arthroplasty: development of a "precentered" total wrist prosthesis. *Orthopedics* **2**(3):245–255 (1979).
9. Swanson, A.B. A flexible implant for replacement of arthritic or destroyed joints in the hand. *Inter-Clin. Inform. Bull.* **6**:16–19 (1966).
10. Goldner, J.L., et al. Metacarpophalangeal joint arthroplasty with silicone-dacron prostheses: six and a half year's experience. *J. Hand Surg.* **2**(3):200–211 (1977).
11. Buechel, F.F., et al. "Floating-socket" total shoulder replacement: anatomical, biomechanical, and surgical rationale. *J. Biomed. Mat. Res.* **12**:89–114 (1978).
12. Swanson, A.B. Implant arthroplasty for the great toe. *Clin. Orthop.* **85**:75–81 (1972).
13. Kampner, S.L. Total joint replacement in bunion surgery. *Orthopedics* **1**(4):275–284 (1978).
14. Bokros, J.C., et al. Prostheses made of carbon. *Chemical Technology* **7**:40–49 (1977).
15. Reswich, J.B., and Mooney, V. *Amputee Clinics* **7**:5 (1975).
16. Bader, K.F., and Curtin, J.W. A successful silicone tendon prosthesis. *Arch. Surg.* **97**:406–411 (1968).
17. Jenkins, D.H.R., et al. Induction of tendon and ligament formation by carbon implants. *J. Bone Joint Surg.* **59-B**(1):53–57 (1977).
18. Helmer, J.D., and Hughes, K.E. Implantable passive artificial muscle. *Trans. Am. Soc. Artif. Int. Organs* **19**:382–384 (1973).

3
Cardiovascular Implants

The development of a number of effective cardiovascular implants over the past 20 years has improved the quality and length of life of people in the industrialized nations of the world where diseases of the heart and blood vessels remain the most common cause of death.

Prosthetic heart valves and electronic pacemakers are the most exciting and successful of these implants. The development and use of artificial heart valves was dependent on the perfection of open heart surgical procedures. The success of these procedures, in turn, depended on the development of heart-lung machines which combine a pump and oxygenator in an extracorporeal circuit in which the patient's blood is bypassed about the heart and lungs during surgery.

Figure 3-1 is a diagrammatic representation of the normal cardio-vascular circulation. As the heart dilates (diastole), oxygenated blood (light) is received in the left side from the lungs via the pulmonary veins, while deoxygenated blood (dark) is received in the right side from the upper body via the superior caval vein and from the lower body via the inferior caval vein. Upon contraction of the heart muscle (systole), the oxygenated blood is ejected from the left ventricle through the aortic valve and is distributed through the body by the arterial system. The pressure in the ventricle forces the mitral valve shut. At the same time, deoxygenated blood is ejected from the right ventricle and travels via the pulmonary artery through the lung where it is oxygenated and, thus, ready to return to the left heart in a continuation of the cycle.

In preparation for open heart surgery an incision is made the full length of the sternum from the manubrium to a point approximately 4 cm inferior to the xiphoid. The sternum is then incised medially with a saw or special knifelike instrument and spread with a large retractor to expose the chest cavity and the heart. To connect the patient to the heart-lung machine, a series of cannulations is performed beginning

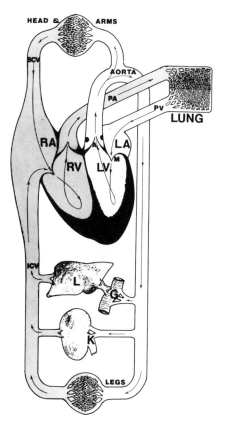

Fig. 3-1. A - aortic valve, M - mitral valve, LA - left atrium, LV - left ventricle, RA - right atrium, RV - right ventricle, ICV - inferior caval vein, SCV - superior caval vein, PA - pulmonary artery, PV - pulmonary veins, K - kidney, G - gut, L - liver.

with the placement of two venous cannulas which are located in the caval veins through incisions made in the right atrium wall (Fig. 3-2). The atrial tissue is snugged around the cannula with a purse string suture to form a seal. By inflating a balloon at the tip of each cannula,* venous blood is prevented from reaching the heart. Instead it is bypassed through the cannulas to the oxygenator of the heart-lung machine, where oxygen is bubbled through it. Oxygenated blood is then pumped back into the patient via the arterial return cannula, from which it enters the aorta and circulates through the arterial system.

---

*Surgitek venous cannul—registered trademark, Medical Engineering Corp., Racine, WI.

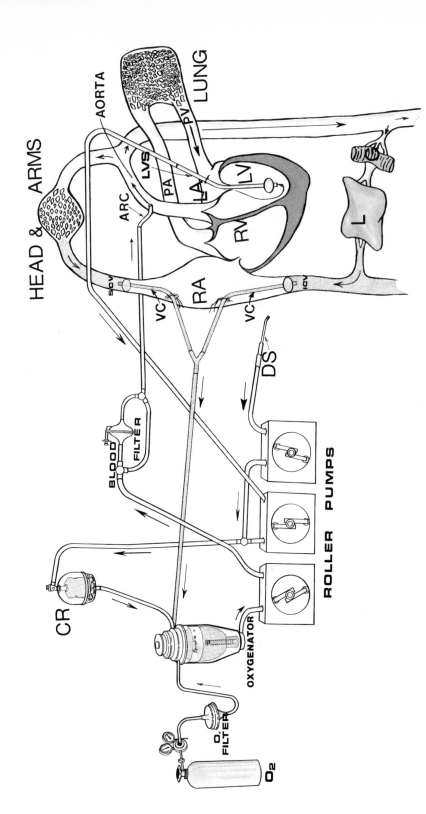

Fig. 3-2. Diagrammatic representation of heart and lung bypass with extracorporeal circulation: ARC-arterial return cannula, VC-venous cannula, LVS-left ventricular sump, CR-cardiotomy reservoir, DS-disposable sucker.

Back pressure on the aortic valve keeps it continually closed and prevents blood from entering the left ventricle. Some blood does leak into the left side of the heart via the pulmonary veins and other blood vessels of the heart. To keep the heart "dry" and prevent distention, a cannula called the left ventricular sump is placed in the left ventricle through an incision often located at the atrial root of one of the pulmonary veins. A balloon on the tip, when inflated, prevents it from slipping out of the ventricle during surgery. The blood which is pumped out is returned to the system. Blood which seeps into the chest cavity from the chest incision is picked up by the sucker and pumped to the cardiotomy reservoir where it is filtered and returned to the system, thus reducing the need for homologous blood.

Figure 3-3 shows a modern bubble type oxygenator. Oxygen and venous blood from the patient enter fittings at the top of the oxygenator where they mix as they spiral down the oxygenator flow way. Oxygen is absorbed by the blood and carbon dioxide is given off, bubbling to the top of the unit where it escapes along with any unused oxygen. The oxygenated blood forms a pool at the base from which it is pumped back to the patient's arterial system. Water connections allow temperature controlled water to be circulated through a spiral tubing heat exchanger to cool the blood before surgery and to heat it back to normal afterward. Cooling of the patient or hypothermia to decrease the metabolism of tissues reduces the need for oxygen; consequently, lower flow rates can be used through the oxygenator. At 30–32° C (about 88° F), which is considered moderate hypothermia, the patient's oxygen requirements are approximately 50% of normal.

The disposable bubble oxygenators are compact, efficient, easy to hook up, and comparatively inexpensive. However, the blood and oxygen are in direct contact as a foam in this type of oxygenator. A degree of damage occurs to the blood; deproteinization, platelet aggregation, and the continuous formation of microbubbles take place at the blood-gas interface.[1,2] The effect of this damage is minor if the patient is on bypass for a couple of hours or less, which covers the majority of uncomplicated cardiac surgical procedures.

For prolonged periods of support, a membrane oxygenator should be used. Oxygen transfer in a membrane oxygenator takes place through a thin gas-permeable membrane. The membrane (which may be silicone rubber[3] microporous Teflon, or polypropylene) acts as the

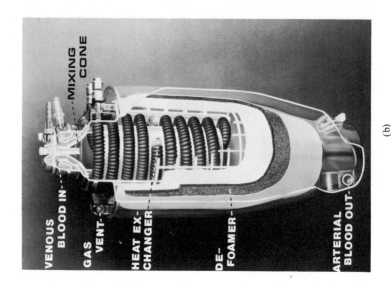

(b)

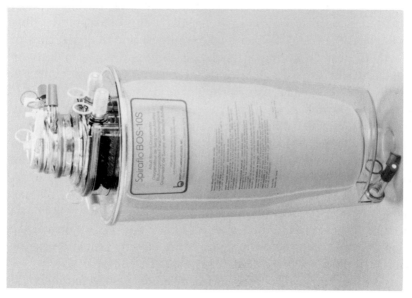

(a)

Fig. 3-3. (a) A modern bubble type oxygenator. (b) Cutaway section. (*Courtesy of Bentley Laboratories, Inc., Irvine, CA*)

interface between a thin layer of blood flowing on one side and oxygen on the other; this reproduces to a degree the process which takes place in the alveoli of the lung and largely eliminates hemolysis, protein depletion, and microbubbles. Patients with acute respiratory failure have been supported successfully on a membrane oxygenator for the extended periods of time necessary for adequate healing and recovery to occur.

VALVES

The human heart beats approximately 35 million times a year to pump millions of gallons of blood through more than 12,000 miles of arteries, capillaries, and veins which make up the circulatory system. During the heart's nonstop activity, constant repair and replacement of tissue take place.

Engineering a device such as a valve to produce a function of the heart presents a monumental challenge. The performance requirements are most severe and must include the following: the materials have to be nonthrombogenic and extremely durable, ideally the moving parts of a valve should resist wearing out over a period of 30–40 years; the design should achieve the least possible turbulence and interference with the flow of blood when open and yet be fully competent when closed; the valve must open and close promptly (less than .05 second) during the appropriate phase of the heart cycle; the surgical insertion of the valve should not be unduly difficult; audible noise which would be disconcerting to the patient should not be produced.

The original work of Hufnagel,* Harken,† and Edwards‡ led to the development and use in the early 1960s of a series of caged ball type of mechanical heart valves which could be placed in the ascending aorta below the coronaries. The subcoronary position of the aortic valve replacement was important for adequate coronary artery perfusion. However, because of the limited space at the point of left ventricular outflow, considerable experimental work was necessary. The original

---

*Dr. Charles A. Hufnagel, Chief of Surgery, Georgetown University Hospital, Washington, D.C., was the first to use a caged ball valve in the descending aorta of a patient.
†Dr. Dwight Emary Harken, Clinical Professor of Surgery Emeritus, Harvard Medical School, Boston, MA.
‡Dr. W. Sterling Edwards, Professor and Chairman of the Department of Surgery and Director of the Cardiothoracic Surgery Division at the University of New Mexico School of Medicine in Albuquerque.

ball valves were made with bulky acrylic cages and hollow acrylic balls. The balls were hollow in order to make them approximately identical in specific gravity to the blood. More recently, the cages have been made of titanium metal and the balls of silicone rubber or pyrolitic carbon coated graphite. Ball valves had reasonable resistance to wear and minimal problems of thrombosis because at each heartbeat the blood completely washed over the ball surface as well as the inner surface of the housing. However, the hemodynamic function could not compare with the normal aortic valve (Fig. 3-4), and the high profile of the cage led to problems where the root of the ascending aorta was narrow and the ball could impinge on its tissues or obstruct flow. When used in the mitral position, the cage often projected over to the ventricular septum causing serious arrhythmias, and the ball itself could displace a considerable volume of blood in a small left ventricle (Fig. 3-5). Despite these disadvantages, many of the ball valves implanted in the 1960s are still functioning, and the principle is still widely used.

Figure 3-6 is representative of the most up-to-date engineering of this type of valve: the Smeloff valve presents the lowest possible profile

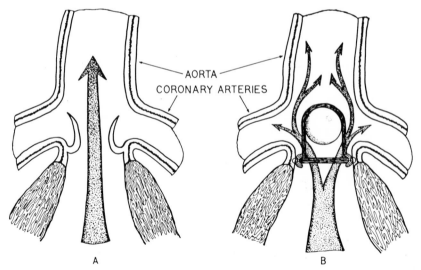

AORTA
CORONARY ARTERIES

A   B

Fig. 3-4. (a) Normal aortic valve; flow completely central, no pressure gradient between ventricle and aorta. (b) Caged ball prosthesis; flow is peripheral and turbulent, and a pressure gradient of about 6 mm Hg can be produced.

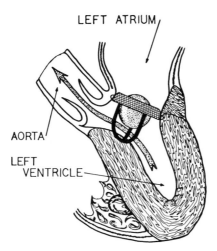

Fig. 3-5. Caged ball valve in mitral position. During systole the ball may be seen as obstructing flow from the left ventricle while the struts are impinging on the ventricular septum.

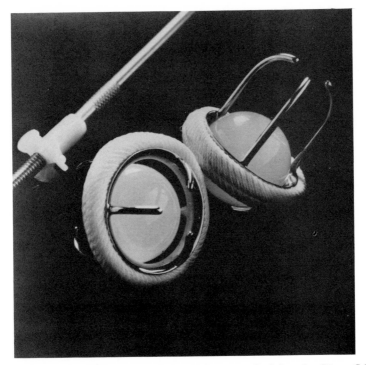

Fig. 3-6. The Smeloff valve. (*Courtesy of Sutter Biomedical, Inc., San Diego, CA*)

for a caged ball type of prosthesis. The double cage is machined from a solid bar of titanium, which totally eliminates attachments and welds, thus obviating strut fracture. The struts do not meet to form an apex; thus turbulence is minimized. The occluder is a specially cured silicone rubber ball which is resistant to lipid absorption. Rather than seat on the orifice, the ball is stopped in the closed position by the entrance struts. The diameters of the ball and of the orifice are nearly equal with just enough clearance (about .1 mm) to allow a slight regurgitation which prevents stasis on the undersurface. The orifice is considerably larger than in the older types of caged ball valves, and wear on the ball is significantly reduced. Long term studies[4,5] of this valve indicate that it has good long term performance.

In an attempt to obviate the space problem of the early caged ball valves, a number of low profile valves were introduced in which caged discs were substituted for the ball. Unfortunately, although their low profile made them more acceptable for use in the mitral position, their hemodynamics were not any better than the caged ball devices (Fig. 3-7).

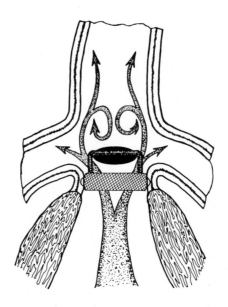

Fig. 3-7. Caged disc valve.

The clinical introduction in 1969 of the Björk-Shiley* and the Lillehei-Kaster† tilting disc valves gave a great boost to the use of heart valve prostheses. The modern versions of these valves combine low profile and a practically unobstructed flow area with very high dependability.

Two Tilting Disc Valves and a Bileaflet Valve

The Björk-Shiley cardiac valve prosthesis (Fig. 3-8), with about a quarter of a million in distribution, is currently the most widely used of all types of heart valve. It was first made with a spherical disc occluder of LTI pyrolitic carbon, shown in the left in Figs. 3-8(b) and (c). The disc has currently been redesigned to a convexo-concave form and the pivot point has been moved downstream; this is illustrated on the right of Figs. 3-8(b) and (c). This development has improved the distribution of flow through the openings on either side of the disc. The improved distribution of flow reduces stasis and thus results in a lower thromboembolic incidence. The valve housing is fabricated of Stellite‡ and the suture ring of Teflon cloth. The disc occluder can rotate within its retaining mechanism and thereby provide longer wear. The disc does not seat tightly on closing, which reduces blood damage; it contains a radiopaque marker to allow postoperative observation of valve movement by fluoroscopy. The Björk-Shiley valve is available in 35 different models and sizes.

The pivoting disc occluder of the Omniscience§ valve shown in Fig. 3-9 is free floating in a low profile integral housing. The occluder is inclined at a 12° angle in the closed position and opens to 80°, placing the leading edge of the occluder tangent to the flow. The valve housing does not contain structural elements which project across the valve orifice and cause turbulent eddies. Consequently, there is a minimum destruction to blood flow with a minimal pressure gradient. Because the disc is free to rotate within the housing during valve function, wear

---

*Dr. Viking Olov Björk, Professor of Thoracic and Cardiovascular Surgery at the Thoracic Surgical Clinic, Karolinska Institute, Stockholm, Sweden.
†Dr. C. Walton Lillehei, Heart Surgery Consultant, St. Paul, MN; former Lewis Aterbury Stimson Professor of Surgery, New York Hospital—Cornell Medical Center.
‡Trademark, Cabot Corp. Kokomo, Ind., 46901.
§Trademark, Medical Inc. Imver Grove Hts., Minn.

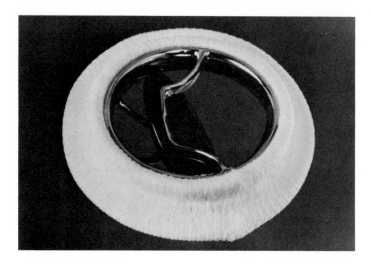

(a)

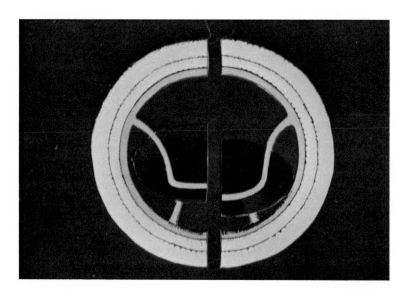

(b)

Fig. 3-8. Björk-Shiley cardiac valve prostheses. (*Courtesy of Shiley Sales Corp., Irvine, CA*)

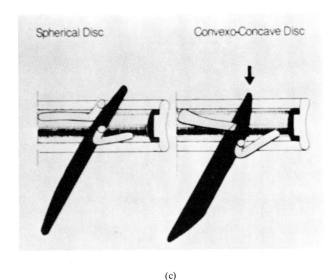

(c)

Fig. 3-8. (Continued)

is distributed evenly. Wear studies indicate a lifetime expectancy for this type of valve in excess of 100 years. The Omni series of heart valves includes the Omniscience which combines a Pyrolite carbon curvilinear occluder within a one-piece titanium housing. A suture ring of seamless polyester knit fabric is rotatable and comes in a number of configurations. The Omnicarbon* models utilize all-Pyrolite carbon construction for both the valve occluder and body. The polyester suture ring is coated with Biolite carbon.

A unique mechanical cardiac valve incorporates a bileaflet principle (Fig. 3-10). This all-pyrolytic carbon valve presents the lowest possible profile, and its developers claim it is superior in effective orifice and nonturbulent flow to other clinically available valves.

The most recently introduced prosthetic valve is the Medtronic Hall-Kaster™ central pivotal disc heart valve Fig. 3-11. (FDA approval to market in the USA was obtained in June 1981). The disc, fabricated of pyrolitic carbon is flat and less than two millimeters thick. A small aperture at its center accommodates an 'S' shaped guide strut which extends from the inner wall of the titanium valve housing toward the

*Trademark, Medical Inc. Imver Grove Hts., Minn.

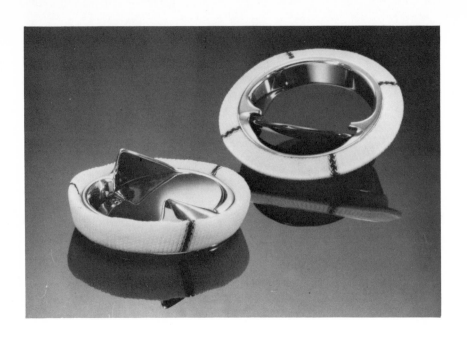

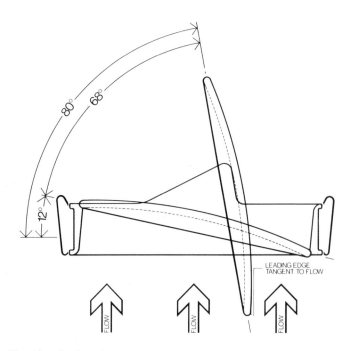

Fig. 3-9. The thin, pivoting disc occluder of the Omniscience valve. (*Courtesy of Medical Incorporated, Inver Grove Heights, MN*)

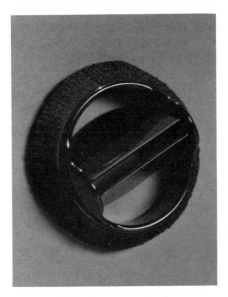

Fig. 3-10. The bileaflet valve. (*Courtesy of St. Jude Medical, Inc., St. Paul, MN*)

central axis of the orifice. The movement of the disc is controlled during the opening and closing movements by the guide strut as illustrated in the lower view of Fig. 3-11. All structural elements such as inflow and outflow pivots as well as the guide strut project into the orifice where they are washed by the blood stream, a design feature which is expected to reduce the incidence of thromboembolism. The outer diameter of the disc is slightly smaller than the diameter of the housing orifice so that in the closed position it rests in a non-wedging manner within the orifice. Also the central section of the guide strut is slightly smaller in diameter than the hole in the center of the disc. The fit of the disc to both the valve orifice and the guide strut allows a slight washing action around its circumference and central aperture, further reducing the problem of thromboembolism. The sewing ring is made of knitted Teflon. Typical specifications for the Medtronic Hall-Kaster™ valves appear in Table 3-1.

Bioprosthetic Valves

At the same time the mechanical heart valves were being developed, some researchers had turned their attention to the use of animal tissue

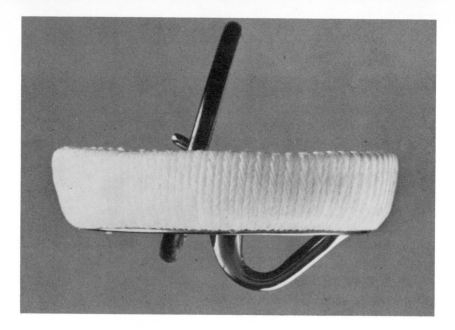

(a)

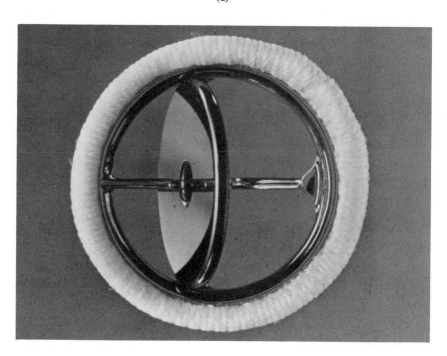

(b)

Fig. 3-11. Hall-Kaster central pivotal disc aortic heart valve. (a) Profile view. (b) Outflow view. (c) Three opening phase sequential movements of the valve. (*Courtesy of Medtronic Blood Systems, Inc. Plymouth, MN.*)

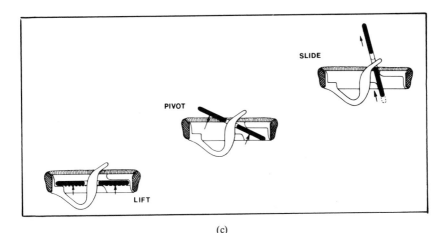

(c)

Fig. 3-11. (Continued)

valves. The valves from both pigs and cows have been used, with pigs' being the most common at this point. Carpentier,* a pioneer in this specialty, in reviewing the history of xenografts[6] states that initially it was hoped they would act as a framework into which the host cells would grow, thus leading to a regeneration of the natural valve. When this failed to happen and progressive degeneration of the xenograft collagen was observed, chemical cross-linking of the collagen with glutaraldehyde was resorted to. The glutaraldehyde-toughened, leathery xenograft was then mounted on a fabric covered stent designed to maintain the anatomical configuration of the cusps and act as a means of attachment.

The resulting bioprosthetic valves more closely duplicate the flow characteristics of the natural valve but, more importantly, they are definitely less thrombogenic than mechanical valves; therefore, anti-coagulant maintenance is not necessary. Where a contraindication to anticoagulants exists, a bioprosthetic valve should be considered, although a series of clinical tests on a mechanical all-pyrolitic carbon valve[7] indicates encouraging results without the use of anticoagulants.

Wear and degeneration of animal tissue valves is inevitable. At the present time, a life span of more than seven to ten years is unpredictable, whereas tests indicate that pyrolitic carbon valves are expected to last a

---

*Dr. Alain Carpentier, Professor of Cardiac Surgery, University of Paris, France.

Table 3-1.

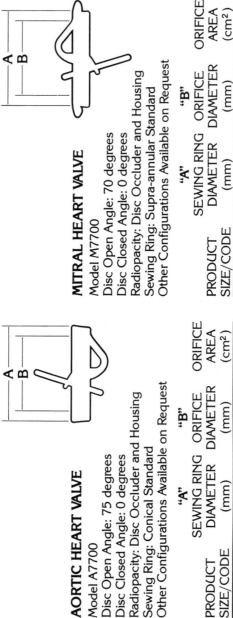

AORTIC HEART VALVE
Model A7700
Disc Open Angle: 75 degrees
Disc Closed Angle: 0 degrees
Radiopacity: Disc Occluder and Housing
Sewing Ring: Conical Standard
Other Configurations Available on Request

PRODUCT SIZE/CODE	"A" SEWING RING DIAMETER (mm)	"B" ORIFICE DIAMETER (mm)	ORIFICE AREA (cm²)
21AHK	21	16	2.01
23AHK	23	18	2.54
25AHK	25	20	3.14
27AHK	27	22	3.80
29AHK	29	24	4.52

MITRAL HEART VALVE
Model M7700
Disc Open Angle: 70 degrees
Disc Closed Angle: 0 degrees
Radiopacity: Disc Occluder and Housing
Sewing Ring: Supra-annular Standard
Other Configurations Available on Request

PRODUCT SIZE/CODE	"A" SEWING RING DIAMETER (mm)	"B" ORIFICE DIAMETER (mm)	ORIFICE AREA (cm²)
23MHK	23	18	2.54
25MHK	25	20	3.14
27MHK	27	22	3.80
29MHK	29	24	4.52
31MHK	31	24	4.52

lifetime. Carpentier feels that the choice lies between an improved quality of life with a bioprosthesis and the greater assurance against a risky reoperation when a mechanical valve is used. Figure 3-12 shows the Ionescu-Shiley trileaflet xenograft valve, fabricated from selected bovine pericardial tissue which has been fixed with glutaraldehyde. The cusps are precisely cut to shape. Three cusps are mounted on a titanium stent covered with Dacron cloth. The fabrication technique produces close uniformity in valve function. Superior hemodynamic characteristics are claimed for this tissue valve.[8]

Figure 3-13 illustrates the intricate steps involved in suturing a Björk-Shiley mitral valve prosthesis to the tissue of the mitral annulus. In Fig. 3-13(A), the valve is held with an insertion tool while nearly two dozen individual sutures are placed downward through the annulus of the resected valve and then through the synthetic fabric sewing ring of the prosthetic valve. The stay sutures placed in each quadrant are utilized for retraction and orientation. In Fig. 3-13(B), the valve has been inserted into the mitral annulus and the individual sutures are being tied. Reinforcing pledges of Teflon felt have been used. Figure

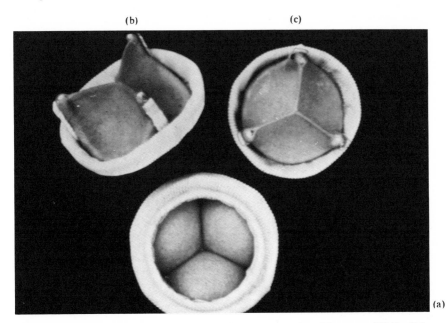

(b)   (c)

(a)

Fig. 3-12. (a) Upstream view: (b) profile view; (c) downstream view. (*Courtesy of Shiley Sales Corp., Irvine, CA*)

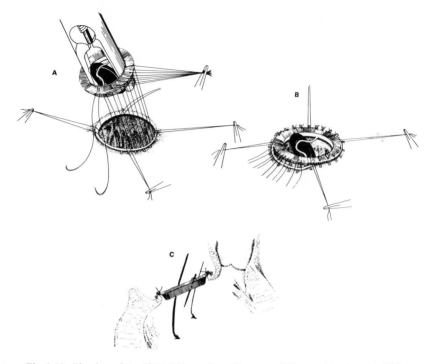

Fig. 3-13. Fixation of the Björk-Shiley valve. (*Courtesy of Derward Lepley, Jr., M.D.*)

3-13(C) shows a side view of the valve prosthesis fixed in place, with the disc oriented so that blood flow into the ventricle is optimized.

Figure 3-14 illustrates the Surgitek Magoven-Cromie* aortic valve prosthesis which incorporates an ingenious mechanical method of fixation. Rotation of the insertion tool activates multiple, curved, alternately opposed needles which emerge from the knit fabric covered base and secure the valve to the annulus. This method of fixation substantially reduces the amount of time required for prosthetic valve installation. The advantage is especially important for poor risk, multiple-valve replacements on elderly patients, on patients with poor cardiac reserve in whom coronary perfusion is especially hazardous because of atherosclerosis, and on patients with an enlarged heart for whom hypothermia is dangerous and adequate coronary perfusion is difficult.

―――――――――

*Registered trademark, Medical Engineering Corp., Racine, WI.

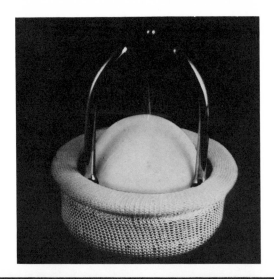

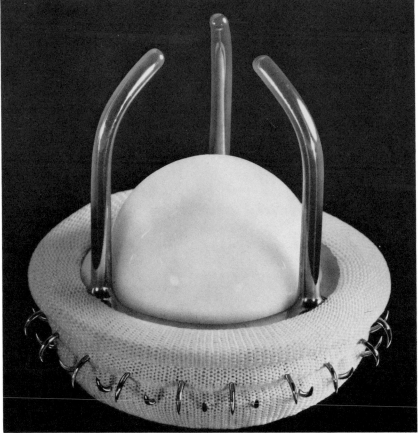

Fig. 3-14. The Surgitek Magovern-Cromie aortic valve prosthesis. (*Courtesy of Medical Engineering Corp., Racine, WI*)

The Total Artificial Heart

Progress in the development of a totally implantable artificial heart has been very gradual. The basic research is costly. The search for long life, flexible materials which are nonthrombogenic has been elusive. A compact dependable power source which can vary the output of an artificial heart, to suit the demand at different degrees of activity, has yet to be introduced.

It appears that the road to success in this endeavor will depend on the experience gained through the development of left ventricular assist

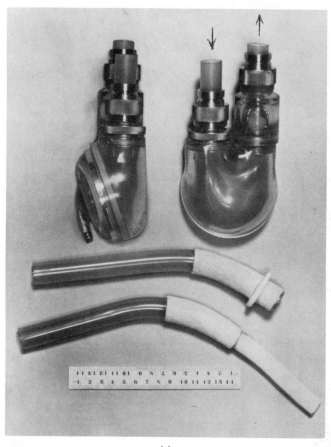

(a)

Fig. 3-15. The left ventricular assist pump from the International Journal of Artificial Organs, Wichtig Edition, Milan, Italy 1979.

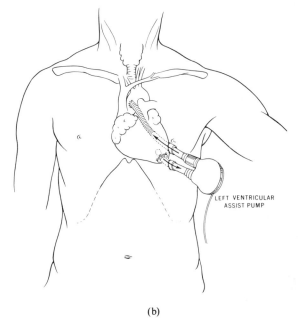

LEFT VENTRICULAR
ASSIST PUMP

(b)

Figure 3-15. (Continued)

devices (LVADs). These are external devices which offer circulatory support to damaged hearts or to hearts which cannot resume their pumping job without temporary aid after surgery. Dr. William S. Pierce heads an interdisciplinary team at the Milton S. Hershey Medical Center of Pennsylvania State University, which has been working to solve the problems of LVADs and the total heart for over a decade. Illustrated in Fig. 3-15(a) is an LVAD which has been used successfully[9] at the Hershey Medical Center; it consists of a flexible segmented polyurethane blood sac and diaphragm within a rigid polycarbonate case. The diaphragm is actuated pneumatically via the connection which can be seen at the lower left. The cannulas for connecting the LVAD to the patient are pictured below the pump; the upper cannula is the inlet, the lower the outlet. Figure 3-15(b) shows how the LVAD is attached to the patient: the Dacron graft section of the inlet cannula is anastomized to the left ventricular apex of the heart, while the Dacron section of the outlet cannula is anastomized to the aorta.

By combining two pumps, one to replace each ventricle, the Hershey Medical Center team has produced a pneumatically operated total heart (Fig. 3-16). Calves which have undergone total heart replacement with this artificial heart have survived for several weeks without respiratory complications; they have eaten well and gained weight throughout the clinical period.[10]

The pneumatic unit powering the total artificial heart is equipped with an automatic control system which is composed of two negative feedback servomechanisms. A servostroke optimizer insures complete filling of the left pump with each beat and changes beat rate in accordance with aortic pressure. A servovariable duration unit insures that left atrial pressure (generally 7 mm Hg) remains within normal limits by varying the length of time air pressure is applied to the right pump during each beat.

Pneumatic power units unfortunately have two great drawbacks. They are large and necessarily external to the body; consequently, a patient's movement would be severely confined. There is also the constant threat of infection at the point at which the air tubes enter the body.

Work is proceding at the Hershey Medical Center on the development of a compact, electrical motor driven system illustrated in Fig. 3-17. A small, brushless dc motor, weighing approximately 1 kg, with pusher plates, actuates the blood pumps mounted on each end. This unit is small enough to fit inside the patient. Initially, it will require a percutaneous electrical lead and will be energized by household power when at rest or by a rechargeable battery pack when wearer is moving about. Eventually a subcutaneous coil will receive power through inductive coupling, thus eliminating any percutaneous attachments.

Vascular Prostheses

The most commonly used vascular prostheses are woven or knit of texturized Dacron or Teflon fibers. Their construction is seamless and they are crimped, which gives them a desirable degree of elasticity with good resistace to kinking or collapse. They are generally available in 15 different diameters ranging from 5 to 35 mm, and are 20 inches long unstretched.

The porosity achieved by the use of fabric for prosthetic grafts is advantageous in that blood permeates the interstices of the fabric,

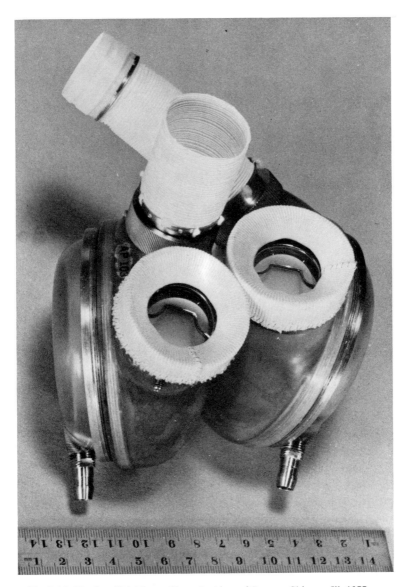

Fig. 3-16. Total artificial heart. From Archives of Surgery Chicago, Ill. 1977.

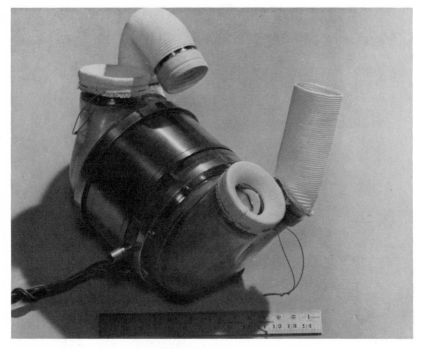

Fig. 3-17. Compact power unit.

clotting occurs, and the formation of an intima begins. Woven grafts by nature of their construction are less porous than knit grafts. They are used when minimal blood loss is desired. Blood loss becomes an important factor if very large grafts are used and/or if the patient has been fully anticoagulated with heparin. Glynn and Williams[11] recommend sealing vascular grafts by soaking them in cryoprecipitate for ten minutes then immersing them in a solution (1000 units/ml) of topical thrombin for ten minutes. A fibrin micronet coagulum is produced which makes the fabric leak proof. The graft is then rinsed with sterile saline and is ready for implantation.

The development of ultra low temperature isotropic carbon (see Chapter 1) allows the coating of vascular grafts with a thin flexible surface of carbon (Fig. 3-18) which is expected to promote the early formation of very thin intima, thus reducing the potential for thrombus formation and reducing the need for anticoagulants.

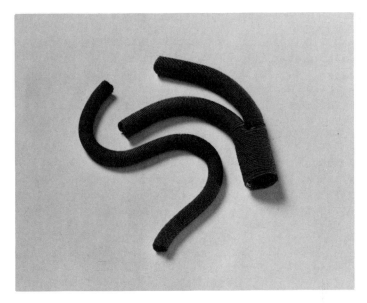

Fig. 3-18. Dacron vascular prosthetic grafts coated with Biolite. (*Courtesy of CarboMedics, Inc. Austin Texas 78752*)

A new type of nonwoven vascular graft is made of expanded polytetrafluoroethylene (PTFE) reinforced by a strong, fine lattice of the same material wound about the exterior (Gore-Tex). Unlike fabric grafts, these neither require preclotting nor unravel when cut, and they have high suture holding power. A limited number have been used with some success as coronary artery grafts where the saphenous vein was not available.

The Pacemaker

The heartbeat is controlled by an electrochemical impulse originating in the sinoatrial (SA) node. This impulse travels via specialized groups of fibers to all the muscle fibers of the atria and ventricles, signaling and timing their contracture. The SA node, which is under the control of the parasympathetic and sympathetic nerves, is called the natural pacemaker. Parasympathetic activity will depress the SA node signals while sympathetic influence will stimulate it.

The signal from the SA node first causes contraction of the muscles of the atria, thereby increasing the volume of blood in the ventricles. The signal impulse is slowed as it passes through the atroventricular (AV) node then moves quickly through the His-Purkinje system to cause contraction of the ventricles and the pumping of the blood to the lungs from the right ventricle and to the body from the left ventricle.

The voltage variations during the electrical stimulation of the heart produce electric fields which may be picked up by a sensitive galvanometer, through electrodes which are placed on the surface of the body, and recorded on a graph. Such a graph is called an electrocardiogram (ECG). A typical normal electrocardiogram is illustrated in Fig. 3-19. The first upward deflection P results from the

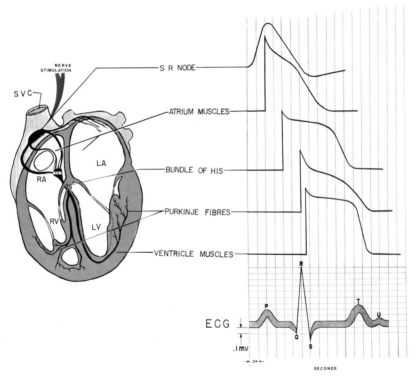

Fig. 3-19. The specialized conduction system of the heart: SA = sinoatrial node, AV = atroventricular node, RA = right atrium, RV = right ventricle, LA = left atrium, LV = left ventricle, ECG = electrocardiogram. Each vertical space of the ECG represents a .1 mV change in voltage; each horizontal space, a .04 second time interval.

contraction of the atria and is known as the atrial complex. The other deflections QRST are all due to the action of the ventricles and are known as the ventricular complex. The number of beats per minute can be calculated by measuring the R-R interval in seconds and dividing in into 60.

When disease, trauma, or congenital defects prevent the stimulating impulses from reaching the ventricles, a condition known as heart block occurs. Ventricular contractions slow from a norm of about 72 beats to 30 beats per minute or lower. At such low rates there is insufficient oxygen supply to the body, and fainting spells are common. Death is usually the eventual result. When heart block occurs, it may be chronic or it may happen only intermittently. Fortunately, modern artificial pacemakers are able to give complete relief from the effects of heart block in most cases.

The concept of electrical stimulation of the heart dates back at least to the late eighteenth century.[12] However, it was not until the 1950s that a strong interest in artificial heart pacing became evident. After restarting a human heart in 1952,[13] Dr. Paul Zoll of Boston made extensive clinical use of pacemakers. His models featured large external electrodes and were operated by alternating current. The first wearable battery operated external pacemaker was developed by Earl Bakken and Medtronic[14] in 1958. In October of that same year, the first implantable pacemaker was used successfully in Sweden. It was designed by two Swedish doctors, Elmquist and Senning, and was powered by a rechargeable battery. It was not until 1960, however, that commercial production of a self-contained implantable pacemaker carrying its own power supply was underway at Medtronic. Improvements in design and reliability of pacemaker devices progressed rapidly in the ensuing years and the number of manufacturers has proliferated. There are now about 20, serving a market estimated to involve the worldwide distribution of about 250,000 units per year. The cost per unit ranges from $2500 to $3000, while the surgery, including hospital services, may add roughly $1500.00.

The implantable pacemaker system consists of a pulse generator, a power source, and an insulated wire lead with an electrode at its tip. The pacemaker is placed under the skin, usually in the upper chest near a shoulder or sometimes in the abdominal wall (Fig. 3-20). From the former position, the lead is introduced through a nearby vein

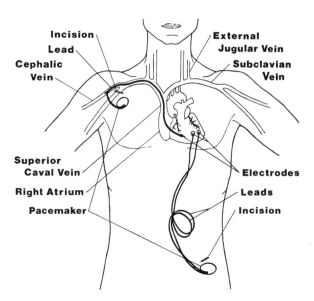

Fig. 3-20. The completely implanted pacemaker placed under the skin in the upper chest or the abdominal wall—both modes are shown.

(transvenous) and, with the aid of a stylet and blood flow, the electrode tip is directed into the right ventricle of the heart (endocardial) where the electrode or electrodes are lodged in the connective tissue. The cephalic vein (CV) is the first choice. However, if it proves to be too small or thrombosed, the subclavian (SV), external jugular (EJ), or internal jugular (IJ) veins might be used. If the upper chest location leads to interference with special activities of the patient such as shooting, the pulse generator may be placed in the abdominal area. The leads must then be carried into the chest (transthoracic) and attached to the outer wall of the heart muscle (myocardial). The pulse generator produces an electric signal which is conveyed through the lead to the heart muscle and, in much the same way as the heart's natural pacemaker, the signals cause rhythmic contraction of the heart muscle.

The pacemaker must be small enough to prevent discomfort to the patient and yet have a power source with a life of several years. It must be effectively sealed against invasion by body fluids which would intereferewith its electronic circuitry. On the other hand, it must be constructed of materials which are compatible with body tissue and fluids. Transvenous leads should be as thin as practical in order to minimize the volume taken up in the vein. They should flex easily and have good flex life. Because of the low signal strength, the electrical resistance of the lead conductor should be minimal, within the necessary mechanical requirement parameters. The electrode also must be a good conductor and resist galvanic corrosion. Platinum-iridium alloys are commonly used for the electrodes, while coiled stainless steel, or cobalt–nickel alloys (Elgiloy) are used in the lead conductors.

The pacemakers produced in the 1960s were powered with zinc-mercury batteries which constituted most of the volume and weight of the pulse generator. Even when manufactured under the most careful conditions, these cells could not be counted on with certainty for more than 24 months of service. Because minute amounts of hydrogen gas are evolved by the zinc-mercury cell, the battery pack could not be sealed hermetically. Pacemakers then were encapsulated in epoxy resin, which both insulated and contained the unit (Fig. 3-21). The epoxy encapsulated pacemakers were often coated with silicone rubber in order to obtain maximum tissue compatibility. Neither of these materials are impermeable, and in some of the early devices, moisture penetrated to the electronic circuitry causing misfunction or rapid depletion of the batteries.

The first nuclear powered pacemakers were implanted in France in 1970 and seemed to be the answer to a power source which would last the life of the patient, since they were estimated to lose one-fifth of their power in ten years. Several thousand of these were implanted during the 1970s. However, the demand for nuclear devices dropped off sharply with the development of lithium power sources. These are solid state cells in which lithium foil is the anode; the cathode may be an iodine or bromine complex, silver chromate, copper sulfide, thionyl chloride, or a mixture of lead iodide and lead sulfide. The lithium-iodine cells are the most widely used.

The lithium power sources can be made smaller and lighter because they have a higher energy density per volume and per weight than mercury-zinc. Since there is no gas evolved during cell discharge, they and the whole pacemaker unit can be hermetically sealed against invasion by moisture and body fluids. Examples of the compact, long lasting pulse generators currently in use can be seen in Fig. 3-22 and 3-23. Initially, the pacemakers pulsed at a fixed rate. Because they

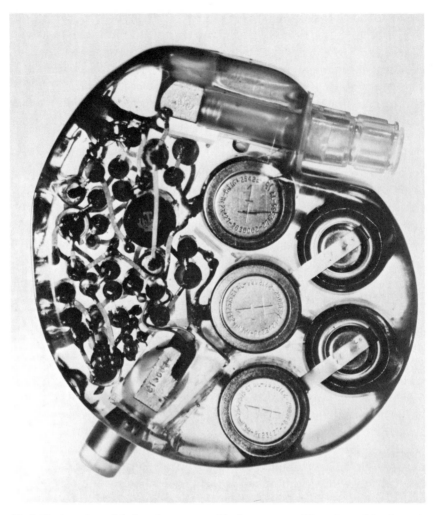

Fig. 3-21. An early model of a pulse generator. The five mercury cell batteries and the electronic circuit components may be seen through the clear cast epoxy in which they were potted. Much larger and heavier than the current models, they weighed over 200 grams and had an estimated effective battery life of 18–24 months, compared with a potential 10-year life for modern lithium batteries. (*Courtesy of Medtronic, Inc., Minneapolis, MN*)

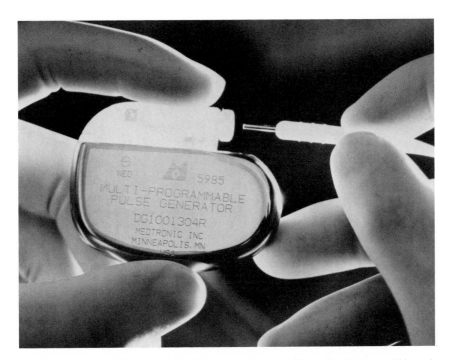

Fig. 3-22. One of today's small dependable pacemakers weighing only 45 grams. Thin and contoured to reduce the implant bulge under the skin, it can be automatically programmed to change the pulse rate, width, and sensitivity to meet the need of the individual patient. (*Courtesy of Medtronic, Inc., Minneapolis, MN*)

could not respond to increased physiological demand and therefore competed with spontaneous heart rhythms, with the potential of causing ventricular fibrillation, more sophisticated pulse generator circuitry was rapidly developed (see Fig. 3-22 and Table 3-2).

The demand pacemaker paces at a preset rate if spontaneous ventricular activity fails to occur within a present period. One ventricular electrode acts as both sensor and stimulator. The heart rate is monitored by selective recognition of the R wave; if an intrinsic ventricular activity of the heart is sensed by the unit, the normal electrical discharge of the pulse generator is inhibited. On the other hand, if the pulse is slow (bradycardia), the R-R interval will exceed a preset limit and the pacemaker will stimulate the ventricle, causing a beat.

The A-V synchronous pacemaker monitors the P wave of the

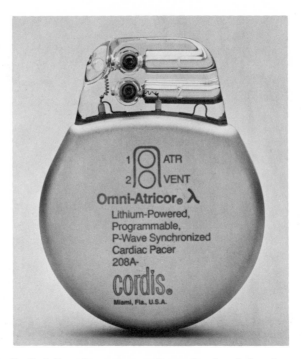

Fig. 3-23. The Cordis A-V synchronous pacemaker synchronizes the heartbeat with the use of two leads, (1) atrial and (2) ventricular, by monitoring the P wave. When atrial and ventricular contractions are thus synchronized, ventricular filling is maximized and cardiac output is increased. The base rate of the pulse generator can be changed by noninvasive electromagnetic pulses from a programmer held against the body directly over the pacemaker. The A-V unit and the noninvasive programmer were pioneered by the Cordis Corporation, Miami, FL.

atrium; consequently, it requires an extra electrode which is fixed in the atrium. Upon detection of a P wave, after a delay of 120 msec, the generator fires a synchronized stimulating impulse via the ventricular electrode. There is no chance of the impulse occurring during the period of ventricular depolarization and causing ventricular fibrillation. If the P wave is not detected, if the rate is too slow, or if atrial fibrillation occurs, the pacemaker will function at a set rate. Normally, the rate will increase automatically in response to increased physiological demand. A-V synchronous pacemakers are necessarily larger, of greater complexity, and more costly than the R wave inhibited type of demand unit. A modern A-V unit is pictured in Fig. 3-23; specifications of the unit are given in Table 3-3.

Table 3-2. Typical Specifications of the Spectrax-SX.*

Pacing rate	70 ppm
Pacing mode	Demand (inhibited)
Rate hysteresis	None
Rate with strong continuous interference	Same as programmed rate
Pulse width at beginning of life (BOL)	0.50 msec
Pulse amplitude (BOL)	5.0 V
Pulse amplitude at end of life (EOL)	3.6 V
Sensitivity	2.5 mV for either polarity of a 40 msec sine^2 wave
Refractory period	325 msec
Power source	Lithium-iodine battery
Maximum available battery capacity	2.1 ahr
Power source depletion indicators (battery output depleted to 2.1 V)	
Pacing rate decrease	10%
Pulse width increase	100%
Power consumption	
Pacing	60 μW
Sensing	30 μW
Pulse energy throughout service life	25 μJ
Rate limit (protective measure)	140 ppm
Size: Height	48 mm (bipolar), 42 mm (unipolar)
Length	59 mm
Body thickness	10 mm
Mass	45 gr
External shield	Titanium (insulative coating on unipolar)
Displacement volume	21 cc (bipolar), 20 cc (unipolar)

*Trademark, Medtronic, Inc., Minneapolis, MN.

The A-V sequential demand pacemaker incorporates dual demand units, one to stimulate the atria, the other the ventricles. Unlike the A-V synchronous pacemaker just described, sensing for both units is ventricular only, through a common QRS detecting circuit. If the R-R interval is sensed to be shorter than the atrial escape interval of the pulse generator, both atrial and ventricular pulses will be inhibited; if the R-R interval exceeds the atrial escape interval, an atrial stimulus is emitted. If the P-R interval is shorter than that set as the A-V sequential interval of the pulse generator, the ventricular stimulus output of the generator will be inhibited; if the P-R interval exceeds the set value, a ventricular stimulus would be emitted. Consequently, the A-V sequential demand pacemaker seems to have overcome the limitations of demand pacemakers, such as A-V disassociation, or of

Table 3.3 Specifications of Cordis A-V Pacemaker.*

	NOMINAL	RANGE
Output current, mA (as programmed)	9 (high)	7–12
	6 (med)	4–8
	4 (low)	2–6
	2 (test)	1–4
Fixed rate, ppm (as programmed)	45	43–49
	47	45–51
	50	48–54
	54	52–58
	65	62–68
	70	68–74
	80	78–85
	90	88–95
Output voltage, V (open circuit)	6.1	6.0–6.4
Sensitivity (+ or −), mV	0.7	0.5–1.0
Pulse duration, msec (at 70 ppm)	0.85	0.90–0.76
Refractory, msec (at 70 ppm)	311	289–326
Maximum synchronized rate	Twice the programmed fixed rate	
Weight, g	96	
Diameter, mm	56	
Thickness, mm	20	
Height, mm	70	
Specific gravity	1.8	

*At 37°C and time of manufacture.

A-V synchronous pacemakers when the natural A-V conduction is not intact. A-V sequential demand pacemakers may be successfully used for the treatment of bradycardia with A-V block,[15] sick sinus syndrome, and other arrhythmias.

Noninvasive Programming of the Pacemaker

Today's pacemaker programmers allow precise control of a broad range of implanted pacemaker functions. These functions can be changed from outside the body through coded electromagnetic impulses transmitted from the programmer to the pulse generator simply by pressing a series of keys. The monitoring of pacer rate may also be done by telephone from the patient's home. A compact transmitter signals the pulse-to-pulse interval over most standard telephone handsets to a receiver at a hospital or physician's office where the pacer rate is automatically displayed and a strip chart recorder produces an ECG tracing.

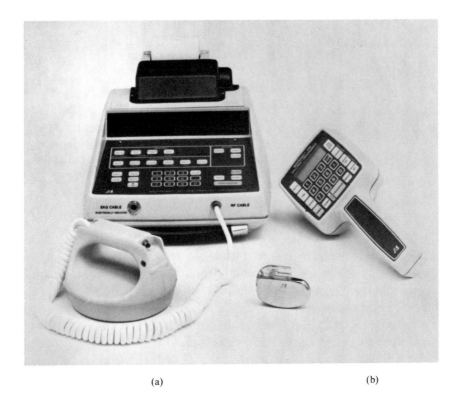

(a)   (b)

Fig. 3-24. Two pacemaker programmers. (*Courtesy of Medtronic, Inc., Minneapolis, MN*)

Figure 3-24(a) shows a line powered, microprocessor equipped device with LED digital display and printout capability. The transmitting head which is placed against the skin opposite the pacemaker during programming can be seen in the lower left of the figure. It is connected to the programmer with a cable. A patient cable will connect ECG skin electrodes on the left-hand side of the programmer. Figure 3-24(b) shows a compact, battery powered, portable device in which the transmitting head is an integral part. The following functions may be programmed:

1. Rate—from 30–130 ppm at 1 ppm intervals
2. Pulse width—.05 from .10–2.00 msec, at 0.1 msec intervals
3. Sensitivity—1.25, 2.50, or 5.00 mV valves
4. Refractory—three refractory periods to pace from the atrium or control preventricular contractions: 220, 325, and 400 msec

5. Hysteresis—rates of 40, 50, or 60 ppm or zero
6. Pulse amplitude—full value (5.0 V) or half value (2.7 V)
7. Pacing modes—demand mode, synchronous mode, or asynchronous mode

The ECG electrodes feed the programmer information on pacemaker rate and pulse width as well as a signal to indicate that the desired program has been received by the pacemaker. The programmers may be used for diagnosis of postimplant changes in a patient's condition, follow-up, and trouble shooting.

Leads

Leads may be unipolar or bipolar. Unipolar leads have a single conductor acting as the cathode, the pulse generator housing being the indifferent pole or anode. Bipolar leads have two conductors, and consequently are generally larger and stiffer than the unipolar. Since both electrodes are in contact with the heart, if there is a failure of one, conversion to a unipolar system can be accomplished without recourse to a complete reimplantation. The increased stiffness may also be an advantage in the reduction of electrode displacements. The unipolar systems, in addition to having a smaller catheter, have increased sensing thresholds; however, increased effectiveness in sensing spontaneous ventricular depolarizations also means that these systems are more sensitive to extraneous electrical phenomena. Because of the size of the electric field produced by the unipolar system, the spikes of the ECG signal may be eight to ten times as high as those emitted from a bipolar system. The posterior side of the unipolar pulse generator housing (the side against the chest wall) must have an insulating coating in order to prevent annoying stimulation of the adjacent muscle tissue by the electrical field.

The installation of the lead may be transvenous endocardial or epicardial (Fig. 3-20). The transvenous procedure is the most widely used (over 90% of all implant cases) because it is a relatively simple, fast approach (averaging about 45 minutes) which can be done under local anesthetic with less surgical risk than the epicardial procedure. Epicardial electrodes originally required a thoracotomy which necessitated general anesthesia. The technique is now somewhat simplified and becoming more popular with the use of sutureless electrodes (Fig.

3-31) and a limited thoracotomy approach. Epicardial implantation is indicated if permanent heart block can be anticipated after heart surgery, in younger patients, and after failure of endocardial pacing.

Despite the popularity of the transvenous lead, the tendency of electrodes to dislodge has been by far the most common of implanted pacemaker complications.[16] Dislodgment is serious in that it can cause loss of sensing and require reoperation to correct its position. Because of this, a number of unique approaches to lead attachment have been introduced over the past few years. Examples of these, as well as electrode design changes to improve stimulation thresholds, are presented in Fig. 3-25 through 3-27 and Table 3-3.

Figure 3-28(a) shows the tip of a porous endocardial electrode. This innovative design addresses the problems of dislodgment and excessive threshold energy rise with a single electrode. Electrodes are constructed of 20 μm platinum-iridium alloy wire, sintered to give a mesh with an

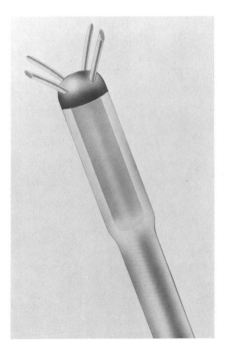

Fig. 3-25. The MIP 2000, first of the special positive fixation mechanisms, consisted of four retractable nylon prongs at the tip of a unipolar pacing lead. (*Courtesy of Vitatron Medical, Dieren, Holland*)

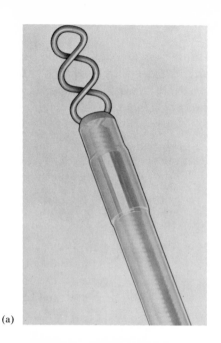

(a)

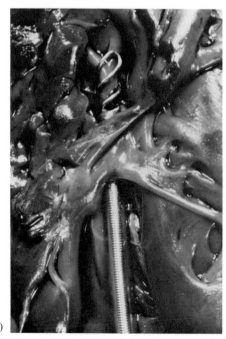

(b)

Fig. 3-26. (a) The Helifix lead, with its helically coiled platinum-iridium alloy tip,* which ensures positive fixation to the heart muscle by two to three clockwise turns. (b) A closeup of the tip showing it anchored to a trabecula of the right ventricle.

---

*Helifix—Vitatron Medical, Dieren, Holland.

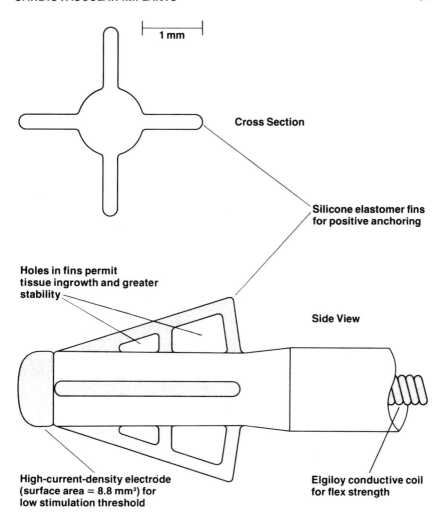

Cross Section

Silicone elastomer fins
for positive anchoring

Holes in fins permit
tissue ingrowth and greater
stability

Side View

High-current-density electrode
(surface area = 8.8 mm²) for
low stimulation threshold

Elgiloy conductive coil
for flex strength

Fig. 3-27. Four small, flexible, silicone rubber fins, with openings to permit tissue ingrowth, help anchor the tip by catching in the trabeculae of the right ventricle. During advancement, the fins fold back against the lead to present a lead tip diameter of only 2.7 mm. This facilitates introduction into the cephalic vein. The small surface area of the electrode effects a low stimulation threshold (see Table 3-3). (*Courtesy of Cordis Corporation, Miami, FL*)

average pore size of 150 μm. The manufacturer claims[17] "(1) fibrotic tissue grows into the structure, thereby providing improved anchoring; (2) a thinner fibrotic capsule is formed around the electrode, which reduces threshold rises and R wave slow rate changes during the electrode maturation period; (3) electrode polarization is reduced since the electrode-electrolyte interface includes the electrode interior,

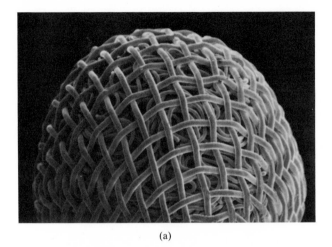

(a)

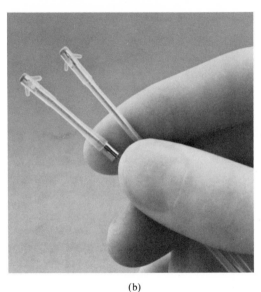

(b)

Fig. 3-28(a). Greatly enlarged photo (approximately ×50) of the tip of a porous endocardial electrode. (b) Lead tips incorporating the porous electrode. (*Courtesy of Cardiac Pacemakers, Inc., St. Paul. MN 55164*)

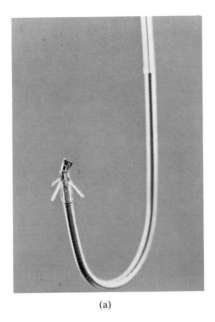

(a)

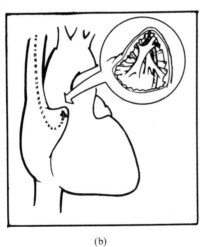

(b)

Fig. 3-29. Atrial pacing lead. (*Courtesy of Medtronic, Inc., Minneapolis, MN*)

Table 3-4. Nominal Dimensions of Cordis Finned Lead*

Lenth	62 cm
Electrode surface area	8.8 mm^2
Conductor material	Elgiloy
Electrode material	Elgiloy
Lead resistance	120 ohms
Electrode diameter	2.3 mm (7 French)
Lead tip diameter with fins folded back	2.7 mm (8 French)
Lead body diameter	2.5 mm (7.5 French)

*Courtesy, of Cordis Corporation, Miami, FL.

instead of just the outside surface area as in solid electrodes. This significantly reduces the electrode source impedance and ultimately results in less R wave attenuation. To a lesser extent, polarization losses during pacing are also reduced." Figure 3-28(b) shows both bipolar and unipolar lead tips incorporating the porous electrode, as well as times for initial fixation.

Figure 3-29(a) illustrates the Medtronic transvenous, tined atrial pacing lead. This has a J shape to allow it to be positioned in the right atrial appendage, shown in Fig. 3-29(b). The tines, located close to the tip of the lead, hook into the trabeculae for electrode retention, as shown in the insert to Fig. 3-29(b). The electrode tip is the ring type illustrated in Fig. 3-30. A stainless steel stylet is placed in the inner lumen of the lead during implantation to reduce the J curvature of the

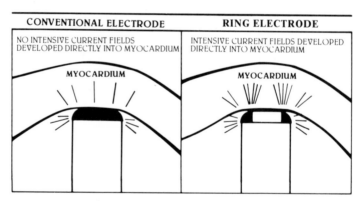

Fig. 3-30. The curved ring electrode presents a high current density at the tissue interface without reducing the total area of the tip. This is in contrast to microtips, which can cause pressure induced trauma. The small electrode surface area (8 mm^2) decreases current transfer during pacing, thereby increasing battery life. (*Courtesy of Medtronic, Inc., Minneapolis, MN*)

lead and provide the required stiffness of maneuvering it into the atrium. The specifications for this lead are given in Table 3-5.

A recent development of the manufacturer has been the use of a poly(ether urethane) elastomer for lead insulation. Tougher and more flex resistant than the silicone rubber insulation formerly used, its thickness can be reduced, thus decreasing the interference with blood flow in the vein. It is also more slippery when wet with blood than silicone, which makes it easier to maneuver in the vein, particularly when two leads are being introduced for dual chamber pacing. This is one of the first long term implant uses of polyurethane. Another noteworthy Medtronic advancement is the use of "drawn brazed strand" for the lead conductor. Normally the alloys used in transvenous leads, which had the greatest stress resistance, had relatively high electrical resistance. The drawn brazed strand conductor consists of a nickel alloy material in a matrix of silver. The electrical resistance has been reduced by a factor of ten. Consequently, less energy is dissipated in the conductor, leaving more available at the electrode-tissue interface. At the same time, the flex life of this new conductor has been increased by a factor of five.

Figure 3-31 and Table 3-6 present an illustration of, and specifications for, the Cordis sutureless epicardial ventricular electrode.* The

---

*U.S. Patent No. 4,066,085.

Table 3-5. Specifications of Medtronic Atrial Pacing Lead.*

Type	Unipolar
Length	53 cm
Body diameter	2.28 mm
Diameter (tines folded)	3.0 mm
Tip electrode diameter	2.16 mm
Electrode surface area	11 mm^2
Electrode material	90% platinum/ 10% iridium
Conductor material	Nickel alloy
Insulation and tine material	Urethane
Number of tines	3
Length of tines	5 mm
Angle of tines to lead body	60°

*Courtesy of Medtronic, Inc., Minneapolis, MN.

Specifications

Lead length . . . . 52 cm
Lead resistance . . . . 95 ± 10 ohms
Electrode
   penetration . . . . 4.8 mm
Electrode length . . . . . . 4.0 mm
Electrode
   surface area† . . . . 10.8 mm²
Electrode
   pad diameter . . . . 1.36 cm
Coil and
   electrode material . . . Elgiloy
Insulating tubing and elec-
   trode pad material . . . Silicone elastomer

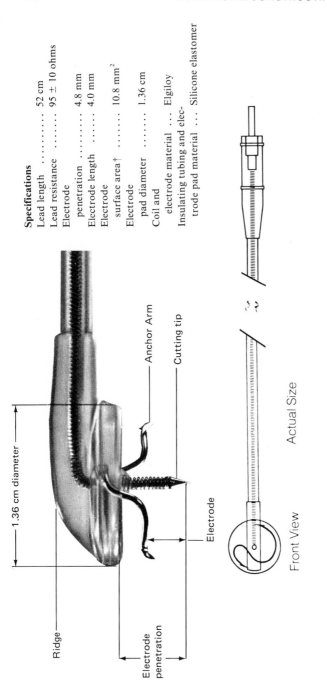

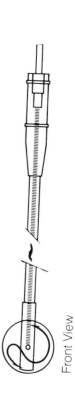

Fig. 3-31. Cordis sutureless epicardial ventricular electrode. (*Courtesy of Cordis Corporation, Miami, FL*)

Table 3-6. Specifications of Cordis Sutureless Epicardial Ventricular Electrode.*

Lead length	52 cm
Lead resistance	95 ± 10 ohms
Electrode penetration	4.8 mm
Electrode length	4.0 mm
Electrode surface area	10.8 mm^2
Electrode pad diameter	1.36 cm
Coil and electrode material	Elgiloy
Insulating tubing and electrode pad material	Silicone elastomer

*Courtesy of Cordis Corporation, Miami, FL.

self-cutting tip eliminates the need for a stab wound. The antitwist anchor arms inhibit accidental dislodgment. The attachment of the electrode to the myocardium is accomplished by pressing the electrode into the heart and twisting clockwise 90°.

Dramatic as implantable pacemaker changes have been since they were introduced around two decades ago, we can expect continuous improvement as the application of ever more sophisticated microprocessor circuitry promises to allow the pacemaker to automatically adjust to the physiological requirements of the human system. Longer-life generators and leads, along with completely trouble-free lead fixation, are other goals toward the realization of a lifetime pacemaker.

An Implant for the Detection and Correction of Ventricular Fibrillation

Ventricular fibrillation is a rapid twitching of the ventricular muscle which prevents coordinated contractions. This is often a fatal condition unless the person is within the reach of a cardiac resuscitation team, with the "crash cart" equipment needed to jerk the patient back to life by applying a high voltage shock to the chest. Now, a new implantable pulse generator with leads directly to the heart can detect fibrillation through a sensor which monitors the heart continuously. Heart failure causes the device to fire a high voltage shock to restore the heartbeat. The device is known as the automatic implantable defibrillator (AID). If one pulse is not effective, it can deliver up to four high voltage shocks at intervals of 15 seconds.

REFERENCES

1. Kessler, J. and Paterson, R. H. The production of microemboli by various blood oxygenators. *Ann. Thor. Surg.* 9:221–228 (1970).
2. Loop, F. D. et al. Continuous detection of microemboli during cardiopulmonary bypass in animals and man. *Circulation* 54, Suppl. 3:111–74–111–78 (1975).
3. Lynch, W. *Handbook of Silicone Rubber Fabrication.* New York: Van Nostrand Reinhold, p. 235, 1978.
4. McHenry, M. M. et al. Longterm survival after single aortic or mitral valve replacement with the present model of Smeloff-Cutter valves. *Journ. Thoracic & Cardiovascular Surgery* 75 (5) 709–715 (May 1978).
5. Brawley, R. et al. Current status of the Beall, Bjork-Shiley, Braunwald-Cutter, Lillehei-Kaster and Smeloff-Cutter cardiac valve prostheseses. *The American Journal of Cardiology* (June 1975).
6. Carpentier, A. From valvular Xenograft to Valvular Bioprosthesis (1965–1967) *Medical Instrumentation*, 11 (2) 98 Mar.–Apr. 1977.
7. Gombrich, P. P. et al. From Concept to Clinical—the St. Jude Medical Bi-Leaflet Pyrolitic Carbon Cardiac Valve. Paper presented at AAMI, 14th Annual Meeting May 20–24, 1979. Las Vegas, Nevada.
8. Ionescu, M. I. and Tandon, A. P. Longterm hemodynamic behaviour of the Ionescu-Shiley Pericardial Xenograft heart valve. *Am. Coll. of Card.* (Mar. 1978).
9. Olsen, E. K. et. al. A Two and One Half Year Clinical Experience with a Mechanical Left Ventricular Assist Pump in the Treatment of Profound Postoperative Heart Failure, *Intern. J. Artificial Organs* 2 (4) 197–206 (1979).
10. Pierce, William S. et al. The artificial heart, *Arch. Surg.* 112, 1430–1438 (Dec. 1977).
11. Glynn, M. F. X. and Williams, W. G. A Technique for preclotting vascular grafts, *Ann. Thoracic Surg.* 29 (2) 182–183 (Feb. 1980).
12. Samet, P. *Cardiac Pacing*, Grune and Stratton, New York, 1973.
13. Smyth, N. P. D. Cardiac Pacing, *Ann. Thor. Surg.* 27 (3) Mar. 1979.
14. Medtronic, Inc. 1977 Annual Report.
15. Berkovits, B. V. A-V Sequential Demand Pacemakers for Treatment of Cardiac Arrhythmias, CVP-Feb/Mar 1980 pp. 29–35.
16. Juncker, David F. Optimizing pacing lead design. *Medical Instrumentation* 13, (5) 289–291 (Sept.–Oct. 1979).
17. Amundson, D. C. et al. The porous endocardial electrode. *Pace* 2:40–50. (Jan-Feb. 1979).

4
Devices in Urology

Next to the brain, the kidney is the most complicated organ of the body. It is not simply a filter, producing urine as a waste product, but a regulator of the internal environment of our bodies. It accomplishes this by monitoring the concentrations of over 30 chemicals in the blood, adjusting them within very narrow limits in order that the blood stream can function most efficiently. The kidney also plays a part in stabilizing blood volume, blood pressure, and the maintenance of proper blood acidity. The complex fluid mechanics of the kidney are not fully understood and consequently their duplication is probably a long way off. The so-called artificial kidney is nothing more than a membrane dialyzer—a form of microfilter.

The Wearable Artificial Kidney

Conventional artificial kidneys are large units installed in centers in which the patient becomes immobilized for five hours, three times a week while hooked up to the machine. Large fluctuations occur in the level of retention products which must be removed from the blood, as well as in the water and salt content of the patient. A wearable artificial kidney (WAK) developed at the Division of Artificial Organs of the University of Utah by Dr. W. J. Kolff and his associates permits daily dialysis and allows the patient to be reasonably mobile during dialysis.[1]

The WAK system is illustrated diagrammatically in Fig. 4-1. The WAK consists of a small, 1.4 m^2, hollow fiber dialyzer connected via a single needle and antiregurgitation valve (ARV) to the patient. As the blood system pump fills, it draws blood from the patient via tube A. The pumping cycle then forces the blood via tube B through the dialyzer and tube C back into the patient. Simultaneously, the dialysate system pump circulates dialysate through the activated charcoal regeneration canister into the dialyzer. A negative pressure in

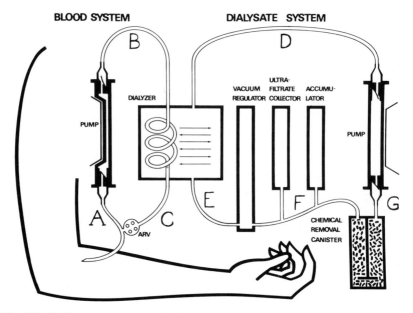

Fig. 4-1. WAK system. (*Courtesy of* University of Utah, Institute for Biomedical Engineering, Division of Artificial Organs, Salt Lake City, Utah).

the dialysate compartment causes the addition of fluid by ultra-filtration. The ultrafiltrate can be vented as required for the water balance of the patient. Dialysate volume runs about 500 ml. The pump originally a double ventricle type as illustrated in Fig. 4-1, has been replaced by a more standard roller pump as illustrated in the close up of the artificial kidney module in Fig. 4-3.

Figure 4-2 shows the wearable module. This module must be connected to a 20-liter dialysate bath approximately two-thirds of the cumulative dialysis treatment time, in order to remove urea. The 20-liter container will fit under the seat of an airplane; it can be carried on the seat of a car while driving or in a boat while fishing. The patient can disconnect from the 20-liter bath in order to move around the house, answer the door, shop, and otherwise have a fair degree of freedom.[2]

Key components of the WAK module are shown in Figs. 4-3 and 4-4. Figure 4-3 illustrates the blood and dialysate roller pump. The pump tubing carrying clear dialysate may be seen in the front section of the pump. The tube carrying blood is behind. Figure 4-4 shows a hollow fiber dialyzation unit—the core of all artificial kidney machines. Blood is circulated through the membrane capillaries of regenerated cellulose, while dialyzing solution is pumped through the polycarbonate housing past the fibers. The hollow fibers act as a semipermeable membrane allowing urea to pass through into the dialyzing solution but retaining the vital large molecule constituents of the blood stream.

Another compact travel dialysis system[3] has been developed at the Department of Medicine, Downstate Medical Center, Brooklyn, NY. This apparatus, illustrated in Fig. 4-5, can be contained in a 21 × 13 × 6 inch aluminum suitcase and weighs 22 lb. Meant for use in guest or

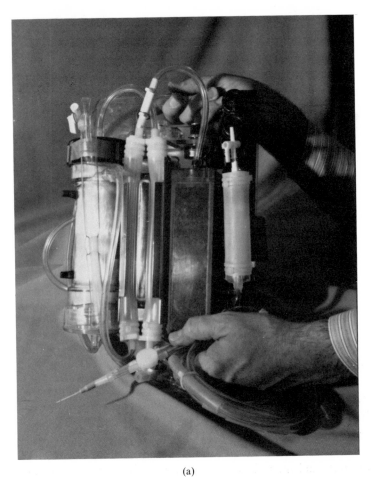

(a)

Fig. 4-2. (a) The original wearable module weighing 3.5 kg (7 3/4 lb). (b) The wearable module strapped to a patient.

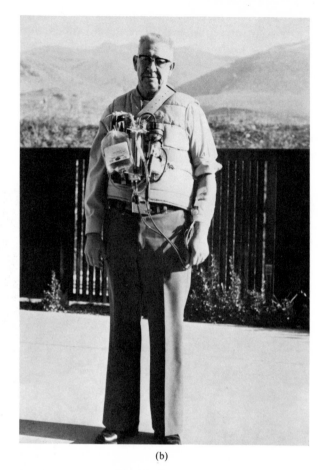

(b)

Fig. 4-2. (Continued)

hotel room, this easily transported home dialysis unit allows the
dialysis patient to take extended trips. Provision for adaption to 220 V
permits European travel. While the delivery and monitoring apparatus
is contained in the suitcase, accessories must be carried in a small,
separate flight bag. This include a hollow fiber dialyzer (Fig. 4-4), the
21-liter collapsible dialysate tanks, packets of dialysate powders,
deionizer, tubing, etc. In preparing the system for use, premeasured
dialysate powders are added to the 21-liter tank. Warm tap water is run
through the deionizer into the tank until it is filled. The dialyzer system
includes an electric heater. The dialysate is circulated until the
temperature and conductivity are normal (97° F) as indicated by the

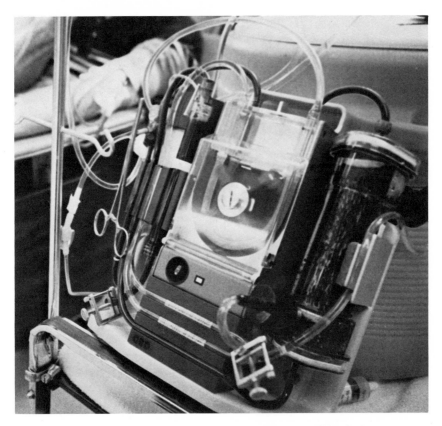

Fig. 4-3. WAK module with the blood and dialysate roller pump visible in the center.

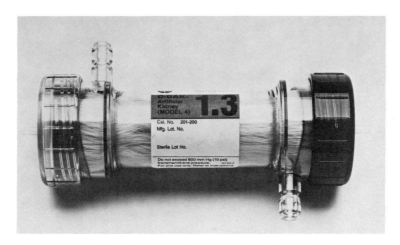

Fig. 4-4. A hollow fiber dialyzation unit. (*Courtesy of Cordis Dow* Corp Miami, Fl.)

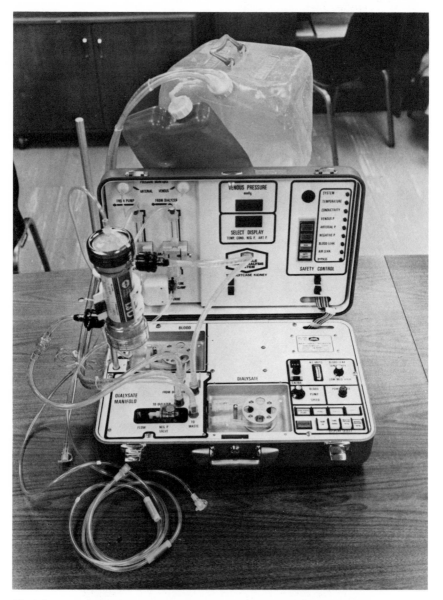

Fig. 4-5. A compact dialysis apparatus showing the hollow fiber dialysate unit (*left*), the dialysate pump (*lower left*), and the collapsible dialysate tank (*top*). Kidney Division Downstate Medical Center Brooklyn, N.Y. 11203

meters. The blood line is then hooked up to the patient and dialysis is begun.

Hemodialysis maintenance sustains approximately 40,000 Americans. The development of compact portable dialysis systems not only allows many of these people greater freedom of action but brings closer the day when an artificial device will fully take over the natural kidney function.

A Silicone Rubber Indwelling Ureteral Stent

Stents are usually used over a short term to provide support after reconstructive surgery or to keep a tubular structure open. However, stenting of the ureter often leads to such long term insertion that the stent could be considered an implant and should be constructed of implant grade materials. One such device is the all silicone rubber Double-J* ureteral stent[4] illustrated in Fig. 4-6. The silicone rubber is soft, flexible, and resists encrustation better than other soft materials. It can be sterilized by autoclaving repeatedly and is an ideal material for this application. As illustrated in Fig. 4-6, the stent provides drainage from the kidney on the left to the bladder. The proximal J is hooked into the lower calix of the kidney, while the distal J is curled in the bladder for retention. The Js are designed to form in opposite directions in order that the distal J curves out into the bladder when in place and does not impinge directly on the bladder mucosa. The stent is supplied in a number of different lengths. Drainage holes are located at 1 cm intervals and markings at 5 cm intervals. It is radiopaque.

The stent is supplied with both ends closed. When it is to be inserted endoscopically from the bladder to the kidney, the distal tip is clipped and a wire stylet is passed the full length, thereby straightening the two Js. A push cather is used to remove the stylet, thus allowing the Js to reform and prevent migration of the stent. If the stent is used during open surgery on a kidney, kidney pelvis, or ureter, a stylet is inserted through one of the drainage holes to straighten an appropriate length of stent. After placing the stent manually so that sufficient length lies within the bladder, the stylet is withdrawn (the J reforms, preventing migration) and, if necessary, the procedure is repeated to pass the stent into the opposite viscus.

---

*Double-J is the registered trademark of Medical Engineering Corp., Racine, WI.

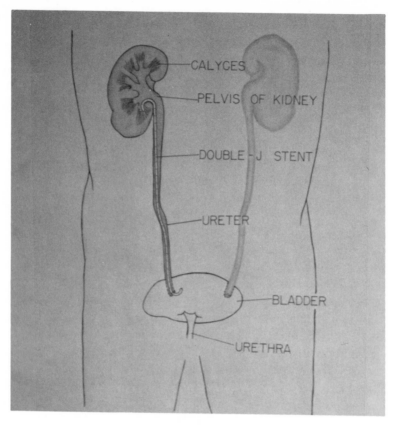

Fig. 4-6. A Double-J ureteral stent.

The Double-J stent has been used successfully for bypassing ureteral obstructions in the elimination of nephrostomy tubes after many cases of open surgery on the kidney, and as an intestinal diversion conduit. There is much less chance of infection than with tubes that pass from the urinary tract out into the external environment. Patients need not be hospitalized, and when it has fulfilled its purpose the stent may be removed, with little discomfort.

Implants for Urinary Incontinence

Urinary incontinence is not an uncommon ailment; it is likely that it affects several million people in the United States. Some forms of incontinence such as stress incontinence (involuntary discharge of urine when coughing or straining) in women with sphincter insufficiency can be corrected surgically.[5] However, paralytic incontinence or incontinence resulting from surgical trauma requires that the afflicted person wear an external collection device or absorbent pads; neither of these is very gratifying to the patient, and they can be accompanied by discomfort and a disagreeable odor.

Several implanted artificial sphincters have been used clinically. The main drawback with these devices, aside from mechanical failure, has been necrosis of the urethra because of the constant pressure of the sphincter cuff.

The best known and most widely used totally implantable systems are produced by American Medical Systems, Minneapolis, MN.[6] In all three models, an inflatable cuff made of pliable silicone rubber encircles the urethra. It is filled with fluid and, when pressurized, occludes the urethra—thereby preventing urinary leakage. Depressurization of the cuff by the patient is accomplished by squeezing a bulb type of pump which is placed in a subcutaneous pocket in the scrotum or labia. Tubing connects the pump to the sphincter cuff and, in one model, to a pressure-regulating balloon reservoir. The reservoir in turn is connected to the cuff through a delay-fill valve. Operation of the pump depressurizes the cuff to allow urination. The excess fluid which has been pumped into the reservoir raises its pressure, which triggers the flow of the fluid back into the cuff. The delay-fill valve controls the rate at which the cuff becomes repressurized. The tendency of the urethra to necrose where it is encircled by the cuff has been reduced somewhat by delaying the filling and pressurizing of the system until some time after surgery—presumably when inflammation of the urethra from surgical trauma has subsided and some revascularization has occurred. The potential for pressure necrosis remains a concern with this type of artificial sphincter.

Patients in wheelchairs are often overweight, which causes penile retraction. There is also some reduction in the size of the penis when regular erections are not experienced. As a result, it becomes increasingly difficult in some cases of urinary incontinence in the male to keep a condom catheter in place. The use of the penile prostheses designed to correct impotence (Chapter 5) has proven advantageous in such cases to keep the catheter in place.[7]

A silicone rubber collar having a D-shaped cross section, implanted just behind the corona of the penis, has also improved condom catheter attachment.[8]

An Implant for the Recovery of Spermatozoa

An increasing number of males who have had a vasectomy as a means of birth control are seeking a reversal—in some cases because of remarriage or loss of a child, or because they may have had a change of heart. The most common method of reversal is through a vasovasotomy, in which the severed ends of the vas deferens are anastomosed.

An uncomplicated procedure in which a prosthetic spermatocele (Fig. 4-7) is used to recover spermatozoa directly from the testis, has been developed by Dr. L. V. Wagenknecht, of West Germany. The prosthesis consists of a small silicone rubber cup having a flange to which Dacron felt stroma is attached.

Lack of spermatozoa in the semen may be an indication of aplasia or long stenosis of the vas deferens. If an epididymal smear indicates a normal production of spermatozoa, implantation of a sperm reservoir can lead to a successful pregnancy by percutaneous aspiration of spermatozoa which are then used to artifically inseminate the partner.

To implant the sperm reservoir, the testicles are exposed by scrotal midline incision. A 5 mm long oval-shaped section of tunica is excised

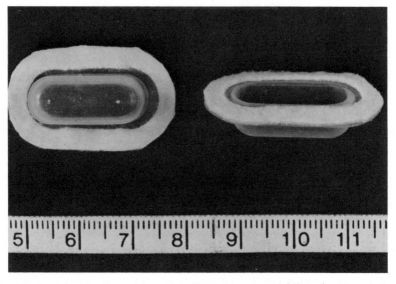

Fig. 4-7. The spermatocele (sperm reservior) implant molded of medical grade silicone rubber. *Courtesy of L. V. Wagenkneckt, M.S., Urology Clinic, University of Hamburg, West Germany.*

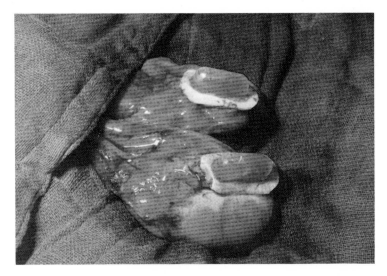

Fig.4-8. Implants sutured to epididymides of the testicles. (*Courtesy of Waldemar Link GmBH. & Co.*, Hamburg, West Germany).

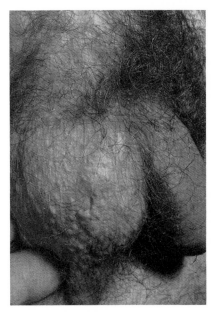

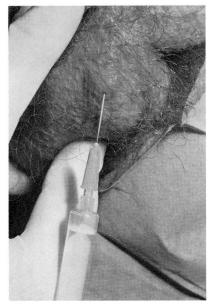

Fig. 4-9. Location of the spermatocele implant is easily identified (*left*). Insertion of needle through the scrotal skin and the silicone rubber wall of the implant allows speedy and painless aspiration of sperm. (*Courtesy of Waldemar Link GmbH. & Co., Hamburg, West Germany*).

from each epididymis. The implants are then sutured over the openings (Fig. 4-8), the testicles are relocated, and the scrotal incision is closed. The implants are readily palpated through the scrotal skin. Percutaneous aspiration is performed using a 12-gauge needle attached to a 2 ml syringe; about 1 ml of material is aspirated (Fig. 4-9).

References

1. Jacobsen, S. C., et al. A wearable artificial kidney: functional description of hardware and clinical results. *Clinical Dialysis and Transplant Forum,* National Kidney Foundation, New York, 1975.
2. Porter, L. How WAK has changed my life. *NAPHT News Research and Technology,* 8 (1975).
3. Briefel, G. R., et al. Field trial of compact travel dialysis system. *J. Dialysis* 1(1) 57–66 (1976).
4. Finney, R. P. Experience with the new Double J ureteral catheter stent. *J. Urol.* **120**:678–681 (1978).
5. Cannon, D. Successful treatment of urinary incontinence. *Contemp. Surg.* **14**:25–41 (1979).
6. Burton, J. H. Development of urethral occlusive techniques for restoration of urinary continence. *Med. Inst.* **11**(4):217–220 (1977).
7. Smith, A. D., et al. Adjunct to treatment in patients with neurogenic bladder. *J. Urol.* **124**:263–264.
8. Finney, R. P. Paper yet to be presented.

5
Implants for the Improvement of Sexual Function

Penile Implants for the Surgical Treatment of Impotence

One of the greatest frustrations experienced by a surprisingly large number of male humans is the inability to achieve an erection. Ancient records, with their multiplicity of weird potions for restoring potency, and the design of crude penile splints or other artifacts to assist in obtaining vaginal penetration are testimony to the fact that this is not a new problem.

Fortunately, with the publication of *Human Sexual Response*, by Dr. William Masters and his associate Dr. Virginia Johnson in 1966, and the wave of articles which have appeared since then, not only in *Playboy* and *Penthouse* but in leading household, business, and news magazines as well as newspapers, there has been a sexual enlightenment which has led many people to discuss their problems frankly and to seek expert professional advice for a solution. Dr. Masters has indicated that as many as 50% of the marriages in America suffer from some degree of clinical sexual inadequacy.[1] Specialists in the field number in the millions the cases of impotence.

Unlike many other mammals, such as the dog which evolved with a bone in its penis, man's erection depends strictly on increased blood flow to the organ set in motion by psychic, auditory, visual, olfactory, or tactile stimulation of the sympathetic and parasympathetic nervous system. It is not surprising then that a large number of cases of impotence are considered to be emotional or psychologic in origin.

Under the capable guidance of Masters and Johnson in their St. Louis institute or through psychotherapy by sex therapists trained in the Masters and Johnson technique, a success rate as high as 80% may be achieved with psychogenic impotence. However, the remaining 20% still represents a large number of people. Added to this are over 50 conditions of an organic nature which cause impotence, the effect generally being irreversible. For example, diabetes affects over one and a half million men in the United States, and the incidence of impotence among them is estimated to approach 50%.[2] There are an estimated 23,000,000 males in the United States suffering from high blood pressure,[3] and many of the antihypertensive drugs used as an effective treatment result in impotence as a side effect. Add to these the not-so-uncommon conditions of iliac artery obstruction,* pelvic or spinal cord trauma, radical prostatectomy for cancer, Peyronie's disease[9] (a permanent hardening of the penis), and priapism (permanent erection requiring irreversible surgery), and there is a large population whose satisfactory genital sex life can be restored only through the use of an implantable prosthetic device.

In some cases it is difficult to determine whether the impotence is psychogenic or organic and truly irreversible. Since normal young adult males have four or five erections during the night while sleeping, techniques have been developed to determine whether the individual actually experiences an erection during his sleep. These techniques involve the use of strain gauges hooked up to a recorder[4] or the attachment of rolled-up tape which unrolls when the penis becomes erect but does not roll back. It can then be measured in the morning and the size of the erection determined. If nocturnal erections are achieved, it can be assumed that the impotence is psychogenic, and a program of psychotherapy can be initiated.

If the use of a prosthesis is indicated, there are two different types of penile implants which have been used with success. They are both manufactured from silicone rubber. The more simple of these is a composite solid rod type which gives a sustained erection. The other is an inflatable type which works with an implanted hydraulic system that allows the penis to be pumped up for intercourse but relaxed to its near normal flaccid state at other times.

A basic knowledge of the penile anatomy and the physiology of the

---

*In some cases of inadequate blood supply, surgical techniques involving bypass by occluded arteries have restored potency.[3] This is a delicate operation, however, and there is some question as to its long term effectiveness. There have been some reports or priapism as a result of this type of therapy.

erection will contribute to an understanding of the way these prostheses work and the technique of their implantation. The major erectile elements of the penis are three cylindrical bodies. Two of these, the corpora cavernosa (singular, corpus cavernosum), lie parallel to each other and just above the third, which contains the urethra (Figs. 5-1 and 5-2). Each cylindrical body is surrounded by a very tough fibrous membrane called the tunica albuginea; other dense fascial layers encapsulate the whole. Near the tip of the penis, or glans, the septum of the tunica albuginea between the corpora cavernosa loses its integrity, and there is direct contact of the erectile tissue of the two otherwise distinct bodies. The distal corpora taper to rather pointed tips which terminate in the midglans. Under the pubic bone, the proximal corpora cavernosa separate to run alongside the ischiopubic rami. At this point they are called the crura (singular, crus). The crura gradually taper down and are attached to the ischial tuberosity (that part of the bony pelvis which can cause a great deal of discomfort when one has to sit for an extended period of time on a hard wooden bench).

The erectile tissue is composed of large venous sinuses which contain little blood when the penis is flaccid. During sexual arousal, stimulation of the autonomic nervous system causes the arterioles to dilate as much

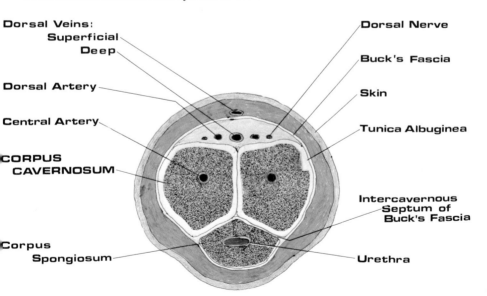

Fig. 5-1. A transverse section through the shaft of the penis about midpoint. The two parallel, cylindrical corpora cavernosa are shown longitudinally in Fig. 5-2.

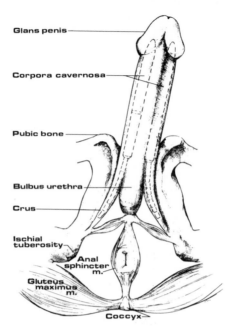

Glans penis

Corpora cavernosa

Pubic bone

Bulbus urethra

Crus

Ischial
tuberosity

Anal
sphincter
m.

Gluteus
maximus
m.

Coccyx

Fig. 5-2. Diagrammatic structure of the penis (perineal view). Position of a pair of solid rod-type of penile implant is illustrated with dotted lines.

as three times their normal size, thus delivering blood to the penis faster than the venous system can take it away. The sinuses become engorged with blood and greatly dilated, thereby causing the erection of the penis. When this phenomenon is irreversibly interfered with because of disease or trauma, surgical implantation of one of the following devices should allow the individual a satisfactory sex life.

The solid prostheses.   The Small-Carrion penile prosthesis (named after the two surgeons who were instrumental in its development) was the first to function with an effectiveness which led to the accepted use of implants for the treatment of irreversible impotence.[5] Simple to implant, it does have the disadvantage that the recipient has a permanent erection and must wear tight fitting shorts to hide the bulge. The relatively new Finney designed[6] Surgitek Flexi-Rod* device (Fig. 5-3), which is rapidly gaining acceptance, is as simple to implant as the Small-Carrion but incorporates a special patented pubic hinge feature†

---

*Trademark, Medical Engineering Corp., Racine, WI.
†U.S. Patent No. 4,066,073.

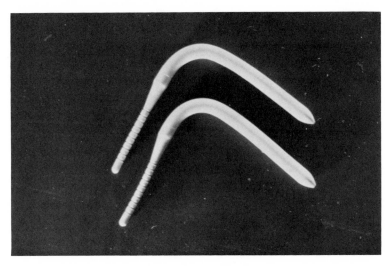

Fig. 5-3. Surgitek Flexi-Rod penile implant. (*Courtesy of Medical Engineering Corp., Racine, WI)*

which allows the penis to lie unobtrusively when not in intercourse (Fig.5-4). This prosthesis is fabricated from four types of biocompatible silicone rubber. A stiff inner rod keeps the shaft of the penis rigid enough to permit natural vaginal penetration and intercourse. The serrated tail section can be cut during surgery to suit the length of the individual crus. When cut at one of the serrations, no sharp edge if left to aggravate the crus tissue. The whole unit is covered with a thick layer of very soft silicone. It is tapered at the distal tip to fit the natural taper of the corpus cavernosum. The Flexi-Rod implant is a simple, popular device for the successful surgical treatment of impotence. An insignificant number of complications have been reported. These implants are available in three diameters (9, 12 and 14 mm) each with seven lengths of stiff section ranging from (70–130 mm).

The solid rod type of penile prostheses are used in pairs, one rod being inserted in each corpus cavernosum. Under general anesthesia, after the tunica albuginea has been exposed by an incision made through the skin and underlying fascia of the shaft of the penis or at the base of the scrotum to reveal the crus, the tunica albuginea is then incised and the spongy erectile tissue of the corpus cavernosum is exposed. Hegar dilators are then used to hollow out the cylindrical shape of the corpus and crus in order that the implant may be inserted easily. The properly sized implants are then put in place, the incisions

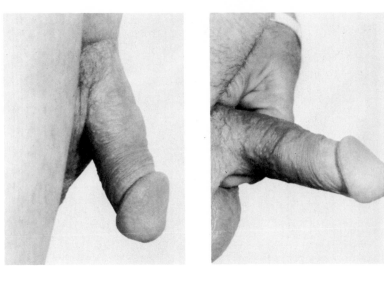

(a)   (b)

Fig. 5-4. (a) A postoperative view after implantation of a pair of Flexi-Rod implants. Note that the hinge section allows the penis to hang normally. (b) For intercourse the penis is manually elevated. Vaginal penetration is no problem. (*Courtesy of Roy P. Finney, M.D., Tampa, FL*)

are sutured, and in approximately four weeks the individual can resume intercourse. The flexible hinge section of this prosthesis allows the penis to hang in a normal way so there is no embarrassing bulge in the clothing, yet it provides enough stability for satisfactory coitus (Fig.5-4). Along with the surgeon's and hospital fees, the cost of this device will range from $1200 to $2000.

The Inflatable Penile Prosthesis.   The inflatable penile prosthesis illustrated in Fig. 5-5 is dependent on a hydraulic system in order to nearly duplicate the action of the normal penis. Two tubular silicone rubber bodies are surgically implanted in the corpora cavernosa in a somewhat similar manner to the solid rods previously described. However, because these tubes require the implantation of a hydraulic fluid reservoir and pump in order to expand them when penile erection is desired, the surgery is considerably more delicate and complicated. The reservoir for the hydraulic fluid is implanted underneath the nectus muscles of the abdomen where it will be protected and where the patient will be unaware of its presence. The pump which is bulb shaped and about the size of a small testicle is placed in the scrotum. The

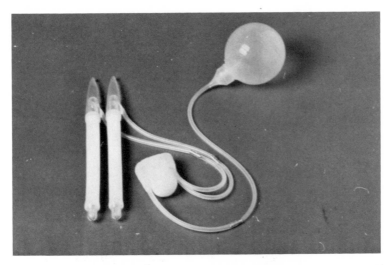

Fig. 5-5. An all-silicone inflatable penile prosthesis, *left*: Two tubes which are implanted in the corpora cavernosa; *center*: the pump which is placed in the scrotum; *upper right*: the reservoir which is implanted behind the abdominal muscle and contains the hydraulic fluid. All three parts are interconnected with silicone rubber tubing. (*Courtesy of American Medical Systems, Inc., Minneapolis, MN*)

reservoir, pump, and erectile tubes are all interconnected with silicone rubber tubing (Fig. 5-5). The hydraulic fluid is biocompatible, isotonic, and x-ray opaque.

Squeezing of the small bulb in the scrotum transfers fluid from the reservoir into the tubes in the corpora cavernosa. Pumping is continued until expansion of the tubes has caused the tunica albuginea to become expanded to the point that it is tense. The penis is then almost as large and hard as with a natural erection (Figs. 5-6 and 5-7). After intercourse, pressure applied to a small valve on one end of the pump bulb returns the fluid from the penis back into the reservoir and allows the penis to become normally flaccid.

Complications with the inflatable type of penile prosthesis include occasional mechanical failure since a fairly elaborate mechanism is involved. Since the introduction of the earliest models, constant improvements have greatly reduced this possibility, and if a component should fail, relatively minor surgery is usually required for replacement of only the defective component. The cost of this device together with the surgeon's fees will range from $5000 to $6000.

The diameter of a penis which lacks adequate girth for the female

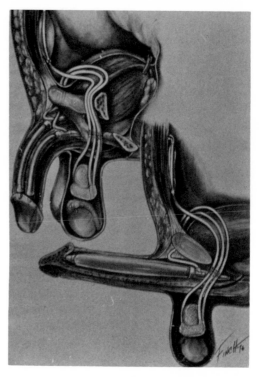

Fig. 5-6. Diagrammatic representation showing location of the inflatable device. (*upper*: penis flaccid; *lower*: penis erect).

partner's satisfaction, can be increased by the implantation of a soft silicone sheath.[8] The sheath is furnished with attachment fabric and encircles the penile shaft between the skin and Buck's fascia.

Thorough evaluation of the patient should be made, preferably by a team of physicians including a psychiatrist, to determine whether there is sufficient emotional stability and realistic attitude for successful achievement of a normal sex life through surgical therapy. Some surgeons have found that initial counseling with the sexual partner has lead to a higher degree of enthusiastic response to the results. However, most reports indicate that the vast majority of recipients and their partners are quite happy with the results—in many cases the salvation of a marriage has been reported. Often the surgeon will discuss the advantages and disadvantages of both types of penile implant and leave the choice to the patient. With their new ability to achieve an

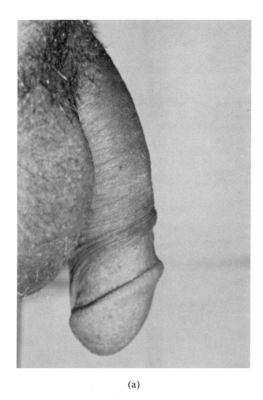

(a)

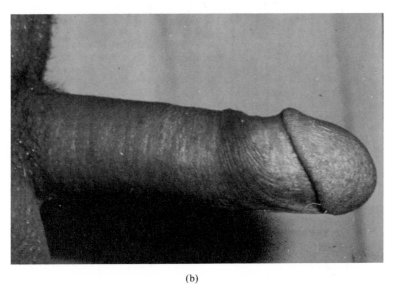

(b)

Fig. 5-7. (a) Postoperative view after the implantation of an inflatable device. (b) Natural looking erection upon inflation by squeezing the pump implanted in the scrotum. Pressure applied to a valve attached to the pump returns the penis to its flaccid condition.

erection, patients who were unable to reach a climax before, may be able to have a climax. Others who could have a climax and ejaculation prior to implantation will retain this ability. Penile implants treat impotence, however, not sterility.

Testicular Prostheses

There are over 30,000 testicles removed surgically in the United States annually because of cancer. There are many cases of undescended testicles, and there are losses resulting from trauma. Although their replacement is aesthetic, testicles are included in this section because they are often a part of sex play.

The popular testicular prostheses are fabricated with a strong silicone rubber outer shell about .4 mm thick filled with a stiffer gel than is used in the breast prosthesis. Testicular implants are available in four sizes (Fig. 5-8) ranging from pediatric to large adult. From the point of view of appearance and feel, these implants present quite a realistic result.

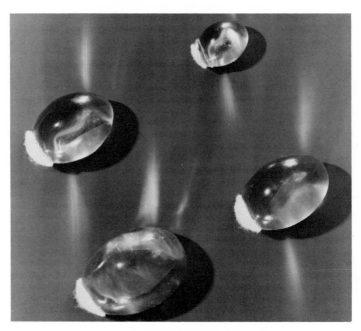

Fig. 5-8. Gel filled testicular prostheses. Dacron felt is applied to one end for tissue ingrowth and attachment. (*Courtesy of Medical Engineering Corp., Racine, WI*)

Total Reconstruction of the Penis

A prosthesis for total construction or reconstruction of the penis has been developed (Fig. 5-9). It is fabricated of a fairly stiff formulation of silicone rubber in the shape of a half-cylinder. A pair of proximal tails are used to stabilize the device through attachment at the pubis. The inner surface surrounds the upper half of the urethra which is surgically constructed with a tubular skin flap—the skin surface being the inner surface. The whole is then covered with another tubular skin flap. Rows of holes in the device improve vascularization between the two graft surfaces. Dacron patches allow tissue ingrowth which assures the fixation of the grafts to the implant. Males who have lost their penis through accidental trauma or surgery due to cancer, those who suffer

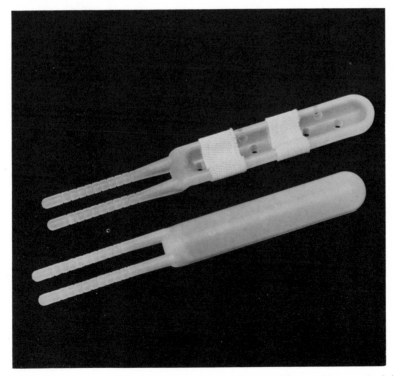

Fig. 5-9. Implant for use in total reconstruction of the penis. This silicone rubber prosthesis is a frame around which the surgeon can construct a realistic looking, functional penis.

from a micropenis condition, or even persons with a gender dysphoria requiring a surgical sex change can attain a satisfying physical relationship with a partner of the opposite sex.

A Stent or Mold for the Construction of a Vagina

Construction of a vagina in the case of its congenital absence or reconstruction after surgical trauma, through the use of a skin graft, requires an indwelling stent (Fig. 5-10). A free skin graft about .5 mm thick may be wrapped around the stent, skin side in. After the edges have been sutured together and excess tissue trimmed, the stent is inserted into a canal which has been dissected halfway between the urethral and the anal orifices to create a skin-lined vagina. The stent is gel filled and easily conforms to the shape of the vagina. It has a retention loop for external anchoring and a central drainage channel; it is available in a range of sizes.

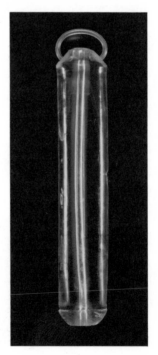

Fig. 5-10. Silicone vaginal stent. (*Courtesy of Medical Engineering Corp., Racine, WI*)

Because of the tendency of a skin graft canal to contract severely in the first three to six months after surgery, the stent will be long dwelling. It can be removed for short periods of time only, for douching or for intercourse (after two months, when complete epithelialization has taken place). Thus the stent must be contoured and pliable to ensure patient comfort and to prevent undue pressure against the urethra and the rectum, which could lead to the creation of a fistula.

REFERENCES

1. *Medical World News,* May 1, 1970.
2. Melman A. The diagnosis and therapy of impotence associated with diabetes, *Sexuality and Disability,* 1 (No. 1) 1978.
3. Page I.H. Hypertension—the fledgling of modern medical practice, *Post-Grad Medicine,* **61,** (1) 203–206, Jan. 1977.
4. Karacan, I. Nocturnal penile tumescence—New diagnostic test for impotence, *Hospital Tribune,* **12** (7) (1978) 15.
5. Small, M. P. *et al.* Small-carrion Penile Prosthesis: New implant for management of impotence, *Urology* **5**:479 (1975).
6. Finney, R. P. New hinged silicone penile implant, *J. Urol.* **118** 585–587 Oct. 1977.
7. Gerstenberger, D. L. et al. Inflatable penile prosthesis, *Urology,* **XIV,** (6) 583–587 Dec. 1979.
8. Finney, R. P. Penile ring and penile sleeve: New prosthetic devices, Paper presented at S.E. section meeting of the American Urological Association, Orlando, FL. March 25/1981.

6
Implants for Vision, Hearing, and Voice

ANATOMY AND PHYSIOLOGY OF THE EYE

The human eyeball is contained in the orbital cavity of the skull where it is best protected from injury. It is surrounded by a membranous sac which isolates it from the fatty tissue of the orbit to allow its free rotation. Six tiny muscles control its movements, allowing an extensive range of sight.

The eye has a lens within it that functions differently from that of a camera: to focus the image of an object at variable distances, the camera lens is moved back and forth; in the eye, the lens is elastic and a ring of muscle surrounding it changes the thickness and thus the focal length of the lens by the application of different degrees of tension.

In two other respects, however, the eye and the camera are somewhat similar. In order to accommodate changes in light intensity, the iris, which is the circular pigmented membrane located in front of the lens and behind the cornea, is equipped with a thin layer of muscle fibers which control the size of the pupil and consequently the amount of light entering the eye. Most of the light striking the retina passes through it. Just as photographic film has a black backing to prevent light which has passed through its sensitive emulsions from being reflected back into them, causing fogging of the picture, the back layer of the retina is pigmented a dark brown and all light unused in imaging in the retina is absorbed by this pigmented layer.

The retina is an extension of the brain via the optic nerve. It is composed of a layer of nerve cell ends. Just above the optic nerve attachment is an area called the central fovea in which the cells are slim, elongated cones; these cells are responsible for the perception of sharp detail as well as for color distinction. Outside this area are rod-shaped cells which are more sensitive than the cones. They provide night vision and allow you to see peripheral motion indistinctly. When the retina receives the light image through an elaborate electrochemical data processing system, not yet fully understood, the image is perceived by the visual cortex located in the lower back section of the brain. If the visual cortex is damaged by a stroke, tumor, or trauma, the sense of sight will be permanently lost. There has been some interesting research done at the University of Utah's Division of Artificial Organs in attempting to stimulate the visual cortex with electronic signals from a miniature TV camera in the hope that some form of perception of objects might allow a blind person to recognize them and be able to move about safely.[1] While initial experiments indicate that there is some possibility of ultimate success with this approach, the complexity of design problems makes this program an exceptionally difficult one.

Cataracts have been the most common cause of visual impairment, especially in the aged. A cataract is the clouding of the lens of the eye resulting from changes in the molecular structure of the collagen which cause it to lose its natural transparency and gradually become opaque. When the loss of vision interferes with the individual's normal activities, the lens must be surgically removed. There are close to 500,000 cataract operations performed each year.

Removal of the clouded lens means that its function must be restored before the individual can see again. There are three ways of accomplishing this. The most common involves the use of extra thick, somewhat unflattering, spectacles. These spectacles have serious optical drawbacks. Side vision is sharply reduced. Clear vision is obtained only through the center of the lens; consequently, it is necessary to turn the head rather than the eyes to see on one side or the other. The apparent size of objects is increased by almost one-third. Therefore, such spectacles cannot be used where a cataract has been removed from one eye because with one normal and one large image, double vision would result.

Contact lenses are superior to spectacles because image size is increased by only one-tenth and side vision is normal. Many people, however, particularly the elderly, are not able to wear contact lenses since their hands are often unsteady. The nuisance of handling contact lenses and keeping them sterile, coupled with instances of allergies, dry eyes, or great discomfort in wearing, has often made them unpopular with cataract patients.

Lens Implants

A procedure which involves replacing the natural lens with a clear, acrylic plastic lens at the time of cataract removal is becoming popular. Because the artificial lens is inside the eye, it never has to be handled or adjusted. The individual often has better vision after the implant surgery than before the cataracts developed. Usually, the person will be able to see well under all conditions with an ordinary pair of bifocal spectacles.

There are a great variety of intraocular lenses (IOLS)[2]. All popular models are fabricated from polymethyl methacrylate (see Fig. 6-1) which, because of its retention of clarity, dimensional stability, and high degree of biocompatibility, is ideal for this application. Various methods of manufacture are used, including injection molding, machining and polishing from cast rods, and compression molding.

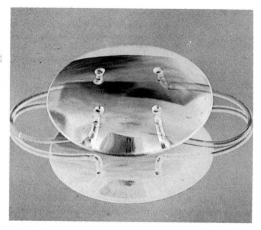

Fig. 6-1.　This iris clip type of intraocular lens, fabricated of clear polymethyl methacrylate plastic, replaces the natural lens that has been removed because of cataracts. Polymethyl methacrylate will not normally cause a tissue reaction. It retains its clarity, transmitting 90–92% light, and will not degenerate. (*Photo Courtesy of Intermedics Intraocular, Inc., Pasadena, CA 91107*)

Some IOLs are designed to be inserted in front of the iris (anterior chamber lens) and some behind (posterior chamber lens). The lenses are stabilized by a great variety of attachments: some are clips of plastic such as polyethylene or nylon; others, of metal such as platinum or titanium. In some cases the clips lie on both anterior and posterior sides of the iris; in others, on one side; still others are designed to be anchored to the iris or sclera with sutures.

The first IOLs were implanted by Harold Ridley in the United Kingdom beginning in 1949. Ridley had observed during World War II that polymethyl methacrylate splinters from aircraft blisters, which had been struck by shrapnel, did not cause an inflammatory tissue reaction when they became lodged in aviators' eyes. This led to his development of the polymethyl methacrylate IOL.

Ridley's IOLs were posterior chamber lenses, and many of them are functioning well today. However, a high percentage of complications and the fact that surgical procedures 30 years ago lacked the fine equipment needed for the extracapsular cataract extraction technique*

---

*When the crystalline lens material is removed, leaving the tough posterior membrane capsule surrounding it intact, it is called extracapsular extraction. When the capsule and the lens within it are removed together, it is called intracapsular extraction. Each has its proponents, and the question of which is the most desirable is highly controversial at this point. Only the availability of long term clinical reports can lead to an objective solution.

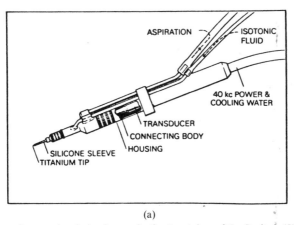

(a)

Fig. 6-2. (a) Lens fragmenting, irrigating, aspirating handpiece of the Cavitron/Kelman Phaco-Emulsifier. (b) Schematic cross section of the handpiece: the transducer vibrates the hollow needle at a resonant frequency of 40,000 Hz. Fig. 6-2(b) published with permission from the *American Journal of Ophthalmology* 67:464–477, 1969.

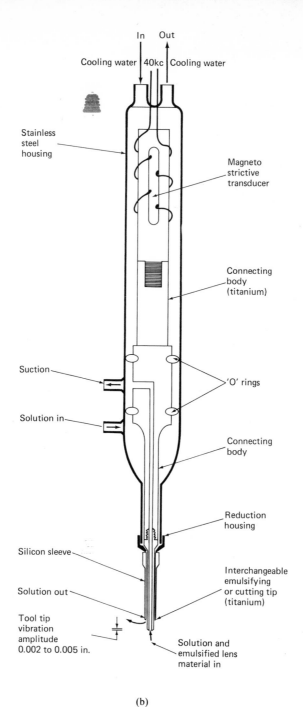

In   Out

Cooling water | 40kc | Cooling water

Stainless
steel
housing

Magneto
strictive
transducer

Connecting
body
(titanium)

Suction

'O' rings

Solution in

Connecting
body

Reduction
housing

Silicon sleeve

Interchangeable
emulsifying
or cutting tip
(titanium)

Solution out

Tool tip
vibration
amplitude
0.002 to 0.005 in.

Solution and
emulsified lens
material in

(b)

Fig. 6-2. (Continued)

124

(necessary for successful posterior chamber implantation of IOLs) led to the general use of anterior chamber implants during the 1950s and 1960s.

In 1969, Dr. Charles D. Kelman of New York City reported on the use of an instrument and technique developed by him for the removal of cataracts[3]. This instrument, known as the Cavitron/Kelman Phaco-Emulsifier Aspirator,† fragments the lens through the ultrasonic vibration of a hollow tip inserted through a minute incision at the corneal-scleral juncture. Suction draws the emulsified lens material into the hollow tip, while an aqueous irrigation solution is introduced into the anterior chamber to replace the aspirated fluid and lens material. The irrigation solution is introduced between the tip and a silicone rubber sleeve which surrounds all but the last millimeter of the tip (Figs. 6.2 through 6.4).

The operation of the Phaco-Emulsifier requires special training and expert microsurgical skill. This technique for the removal of cataracts offers the benefit of a much smaller incision with resultant faster healing and return of the patient to full activity in a day or two. It has also contributed to a growing popularization of the posterior chamber lens because of the improved ease of extracapsular extraction.

It has been claimed by the practitioners of extrascapsular techniques that the resultant retention of the posterior membrane as a barrier between the vitreous and anterior chambers is an advantage in that it keeps the vitreous intact, reduces the chances of cystoid macular edema, lowers the incidence of retinal tears, and makes aphakic penetrating keratoplasty safer and technically easier.[4]

Dr. Norman Jaffe, a well-known opthalmologist of Miami Beach, Florida has had very extensive experience with intraocular lens implantation. He cites the following advantages and disadvantages of posterior chamber vs anterior chamber lenses.[4] Advantages of the posterior chamber lens include the following:

1. Best physiologic position—Its position more closely parallels that of the crystalline lens than other intraocular lenses.
2. Greatest separation from the cornea and anterior chamber angle—This reduces the likelihood of corneal edema or the uveitis, glaucoma, hyphema syndrome.

---

† Registered trademark, Cavitron Surgical Systems, Division of Syntel, Inc., Irvine, CA 92714.

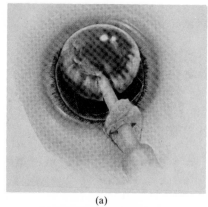

(a)

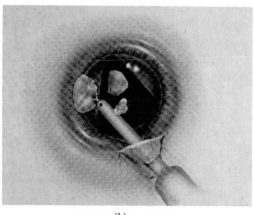

(b)

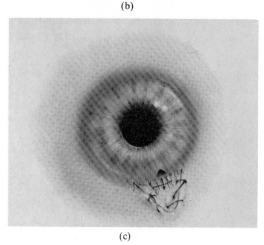

(c)

Fig. 6-3. (a) The opaque lens nucleus has been surgically prolapsed into the anterior chamber of the eye and the tip of the Phaco-Emulsifier introduced through a small 2–3 mm incision to engage the lens. (b) Lens nucleus being fragmented by the ultrasonic vibration of the tip; the fragments are being aspirated simultaneously through the hollow tip. (c) Conclusion of the procedure: because of the very small surgical incision, excellent wound closure during healing is assured and healing is rapid. The patient usually can return to normal activity the next day. (*Courtesy of Cavitron Surgical Systems*)

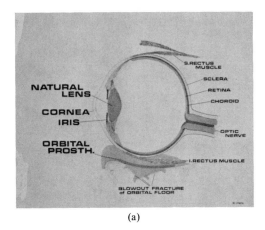

(a)

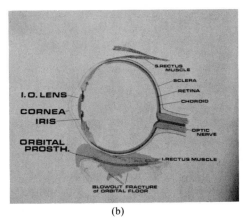

(b)

Fig. 6-4. (a) Structure of normal human eye (except for repair of orbital floor). (b) After removal of cataract and implantation of acrylic intraocular lens (IOL).

3. Easiest intraocular lens to insert without making contact with the cornea.
4. Free mobility of the pupil—This is a significant advantage because it permits adequate dilation of the pupil for ophthalmoscopic examination. The pupil responds physiologically in conditions of light and dark.
5. Cosmesis—The pupil appears normal. This is a minor advantage.

6. Less pseudophakodonesis—The importance of this in preventing inflammation and cystoid macular edema has not been proven.
7. Less danger of corneal contact with postoperative abnormalities of anterior chamber depth—This is a significant advantage.
8. Less glitter, dazzle, flutter, and edge glare—Patients with pre-pupillary lenses occasionally complain of reflections, image duplication, halos, and the like. This has been virtually eliminated with posterior chamber lenses.

Disadvantages of the posterior chamber lens include the following:

1. No long-term results—No long-term experience, favorable or unfavorable, exists of the intraocular tolerance of posterior chamber lenses.
2. The Shearing posterior chamber lens depends on the capsule and ciliary sulcus for fixation—This may prove to be inadequate in the long run.
3. The Pearce posterior chamber lens requires a fixation suture—This complicates the procedure.
4. Can only be used with an extracapsular cataract extraction—This is a significant disadvantage for those who must radically change their method of cataract surgery and for those who are not convinced of the advantage of the extracapsular cataract extraction.
5. Impingement on ciliary body structures—This particularly involves the Shearing lens. If it is intended that the two loops of the implant rest in the ciliary sulcus, the insertion must be considered a blind procedure. The long-term tolerance of ciliary body structures of contact with the loops is unknown.
6. Difficult to remove—The Shearing lens is probably the most difficult implant to remove. The Pearce lens can be removed more easily but still with greater difficulty than other types of intraocular lenses.

Advantages of the anterior chamber angle-supported lens include the following:

1. Ease of insertion—The ease of insertion is comparable to that of the Shearing lens. However, as stated previously with the

Shearing lens, the insertion is somewhat of a blind procedure because the surgeon cannot visualize the exact location in the anterior chamber angle where the ends of the haptic are supposed to be placed.

2. Dilatable pupil—This advantage is significant and has been previously discussed.

3. Least pseudophakodonesis—When properly inserted, this type of implant gives the least pseudophakodonesis of all the types of implants. The advantage of this is still unknown.

4. Little risk if dislocation—This is a true advantage shown clinically.

5. Cosmesis—The pupil appears to be nearly normal. Occasionally, there is an oval-shaped pupil in the direction of the long axis of the implant. This is not a significant advantage.

6. Best intraocular lens for secondary implantation—This is one of its most important advantages. However, it should not be considered a stimulus for a more liberal interpretation of the indication for secondary lens implantation.

7. Can be used with either an intra- or extracapsular cataract extraction—This is a significant advantage because it requires the surgeon to change his method of cataract extraction.

Disadvantages of the anterior chamber angle-supported lens include the following:

1. Dimensions of the implant are critical—There are significant disadvantages to a too-short or too-long implant. Therefore, dependence on accurate estimation of the width of the anterior chamber and the manufacturer's designation of the length of the implant is a disadvantage.

2. Controversy over manufacture—This implant has created more controversy over quality of manufacture than any other implant. The sharp edges of injection molded lenses in particular have resulted in serious problems.

3. Sputtering hyphema—Ellingson reported the association of uveitis, glaucoma, and hyphema. This has resulted in the removal of many of these lens implants after successful surgery, which appears to be related to the quality of the manufactured product. This complication is rare with other types of intraocular lenses.

4. Placement is a blind procedure—It is impossible to visualize the structures of the anterior chamber angle where the ends of the haptics are intended to insert.
5. Eyes are tender—This complication tends to diminish with time but it may be annoying to some patients. This does not occur with other intraocular lenses.
6. Late uveitis—This is usually not difficult to manage and it also occurs with other intraocular lenses.
7. Few long-term results—With the exception of Choyce, there have been few long-term clinical studies of anterior chamber angle-supported lenses.

IRIS OR IRIS AND CAPSULE SUPPORTED LENSES

Epstein was the first to use an iris-supported lens. There are now many iris or iris and capsule supported intraocular lenses. Among these are the Binkhorst iris clip, Binkhorst iridocapsular, Worst Medallion, Worst vertical clip, Fyodorov-Binkhorst, Fyodorov Sputnik, and Copeland-Epstein.

Advantages of the iris or iris and capsule supported lens include the following:

1. Angle structures are spared—The ends of the haptics are separated by a comfortable distance from the anterior chamber angle structures.
2. Widely separated from the cornea—There is less danger of corneal touch than with an anterior chamber angle-supported lens but much greater than with a posterior chamber lens.
3. Consistency of manufactured product—Small changes in model design by different manufacturers seem to have little influence on the safety of this type of lens.
4. Long history of good ocular tolerance—This lens has probably had the greatest number of observed series of any type of lens implant. The long-range tolerance seems to be satisfactory at this time.
5. No ocular tenderness—There is no tenderness of the eyeball on palpation.
6. May be used with an intra- or extracapsular cataract extraction—This advantage is shared with the anterior chamber angle-supported lens.

Disadvantages of the iris or iris and capsule supported lens include the following:

1. Iris fixation required—With the exception of the Copeland lens and possibly the Fyodorov-Binkhorst lens, this type of lens must have some form of fixation to the iris when used with an intracapsular cataract extraction. This makes the surgery more complex.
2. Capsule fixation required—Most of the lenses in this group that are used with an extracapsular cataract extraction require some form of capsule fixation. This is not always achieved.
3. Dislocations more frequent—These lens implants have the highest frequency of dislocation of any type of implant. Iris or capsule fixation does not ensure against a dislocation. One or more haptic elements of the implant may dislocate. Contact with the cornea is not infrequent. Those implants in this group that are not fixated with a suture present the additional risk of dislocation into the vitreous.
4. The easier to insert lens implants cause more complications—The Copeland and Fyodorov-Binkhorst implants that are not sutured to the iris often cause more complications. The more sophisticated implants in this group are more difficult to insert but are associated with less postoperative complications.
5. Pseudophakodonesis—These lenses cause the greatest amount of pseudophakodonesis. They are supported by the iris, which is a movable part of the eye and therefore their additional weight increases this motion.
6. Square pupil—This is an unimportant cosmetic blemish that is usually not obvious.
7. Difficulty in dilating the pupil—Iris synechiae to the implant often prevent adequate dilation for ophthalmoscopic examination.

Jaffe's concludes "that there is little difference in final visual acuity regardless of which implant or cataract technique is used." Jaffe N., The changing scene of Intraocular Implant Surgery Published with permission from the *American Journal of Ophthalmology* **88**:419–828, 1979.

While lens implant surgery may take less than one hour under local anesthetic and the patient can usually leave the hospital the next day, it is a delicate operation and it is not without serious risk. Nevertheless, when an elderly person has the opportunity of seeing clearly again, without the drawbacks of external devices, the risk seems well worth taking.

Implants for Treatment of Fracture of the Orbital Floor

Because the eye is contained within the bony orbit, the force of a blow to the eye from an object such as a ball or a fist can be transmitted hydraulically to the walls of the orbit. The floor or lower section is quite thin and under stress will sometimes fracture, breaking downward into the maxillary sinus (Fig. 6-5). When this happens, the eyeball can drop into the space created by the fracture, causing diplopia or double vision, or the inferior muscles may become entrapped in the break, thus limiting eye movement. Past methods of treating an orbital floor fracture included reduction of the fracture through a packing inserted in the sinus cavity. This necessitated removal of the packing after the

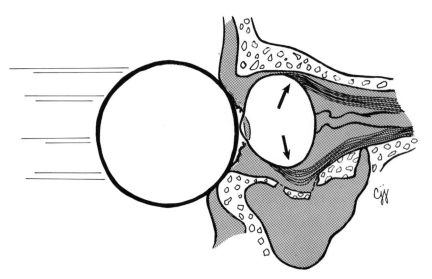

Fig. 6-5. Blow-out fracture of the orbital floor occurs when an object such as a ball strikes the eye and the force is distributed hydraulically by compression of the eyeball and the orbital fat. Repair of the fracture with an orbital implant may be seen in Fig. 6-4.

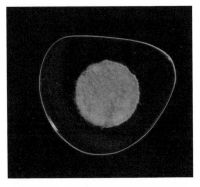 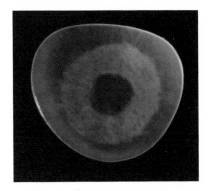

Fig. 6-6. Spherically shaped premolded orbital floor implants of silicone rubber, bonded on Dacron felt in various patterns for tissue ingrowth and attachment. (*Photo Courtesy of Medical Engineering Corporation*)

orbital floor bones had set. Subsequent closing and healing of the surgical opening into the sinus were additional steps involved.

A popular treatment today involves implantation of a spherical segment of silicone rubber (Fig. 6-6), Teflon, or tantalum mesh, which becomes a permanent support for the eyeball. An incision is made through the lower eyelid, and the tunica covering the rectus muscle is dissected from the orbital fat. The orbital floor implant is trimmed to suit, particular care being taken to provide a generous notch in the area of the optic nerve. When the implant is slipped into place, the eyeball will be raised to its normal level. Reduction of the fracture is ignored— it is left to heal as is. A wire suture is often used to attach the implant to the orbital bone anteriorly to keep it from slipping forward and causing protrusion of the lower eyelid. Location of the orbital implant may be seen in Fig. 6.4.

THE EAR

If Beethoven were alive today it is likely that a large part of his lost hearing could be restored through implant surgery. A common cause of deafness is the sclerotic fixation of the small bones of the middle ear. Beethoven is believed to have suffered this form of deafness. Through expert microsurgery and the use of minute implants (some not over 2 mm in diameter) to replace degenerated moving parts of the middle ear, satisfactory hearing can be achieved.

The structure of the human ear includes three main parts: the outer ear, the middle ear, and the inner ear (Fig. 6-7). The outer ear collects sounds which are conveyed through the auditory canal to the eardrum (tympanic membrane) causing it to vibrate. The vibrations of the eardrum are, in turn, transmitted and increased in pressure by the lever action of the three bones of the middle ear to a thin membrane of the inner ear called the oval window. In the inner ear, the transmitted energy is converted into nerve impulses which are conducted to the auditory cortex of the brain where they are converted into sensations of pitch, quality, and loudness and also into information about the direction or origin of the sound. The inner ear (Fig. 6-10) also embodies three semicircular canals which are responsible for the sense of balance.

All of this intricate, sensitive, and delicate mechanism is housed within a very small space of the temporal bones* at their thickest and hardest section, where maximum protection is attained.

---

*The two irregular bones which form part of the lateral surfaces and base of the skull.

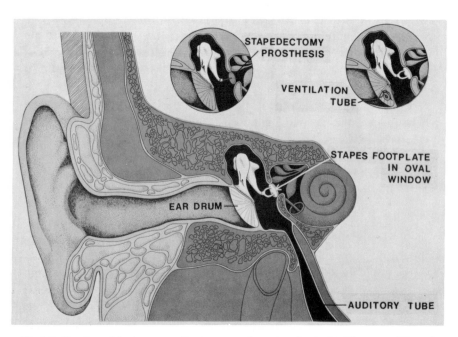

Fig. 6-7. Structure of the human ear (*inset:* commonly used ear implants). (*Courtesy of Xomed, Inc., Jacksonville, FL*)

Inplants for the Middle Ear

On the inner surface of the eardrum, the first of the three middle ear bones known as the hammer (malleus) is attached. This articulates the anvil (incus) which is connected to the stirrup (stapes) which transmits the sound vibrations to the oval window.

Otosclerosis is the formation of spongy bone in the labyrinth of the middle ear which gradually limits the movement of the bones of the middle ear and leads to deafness. A common method of correcting this condition includes the surgical removal of the stapes bone and its replacement with a stapedectomy prosthesis (Figs. 6–7 and 6–8). There are many designs of stapedectomy prostheses; materials used in their construction include Teflon (solid or porous), stainless steel, platinum, and Gelfoam.*

When removal of all three ossicular bones becomes necessary, a total ossicular implant will be used to connect the inner surface of the eardrum directly to the oval window. In addition to the other materials mentioned, Proplast has been used successfully in this application.[7]

Secretory otitis media is an inflammation of the middle ear, accompanied by inadequate aeration or drainage via the eustachian tube. Tympanotomy ventilation tubes (Figs. 6–7 and 6–9) are the preferred method of treatment.[8] As in the case of the stapedectomy prostheses there are many designs of middle ear ventilation tubes.[9]

Cochlear Prosthesis

Conversion of the vibrations transmitted by the stapes to the oval window, into electrochemical nerve signals to the brain, takes place in the cochlea—a hard snail-like structure of the inner ear (Fig. 6-10). The spiral tube of the cochlea is filled with fluid and is divided in two along its length by a thin, tough membrane called the basilar membrane. Thousands of fine hair cell nerve structures stand up from the membrane and synapse nerve fibers which run into the auditory nerve. Each oscillation of the oval window produces a to-and-fro movement of the fluid in the cohlea which causes a wave to travel along the basilar membrane.[10] The movement of the membrane bends certain of the hair cells, which then fire off impulses to the brain. The traveling wave

---

*Gelfoam—regular trademark, Upjohn Co. Torrance, CA 90503

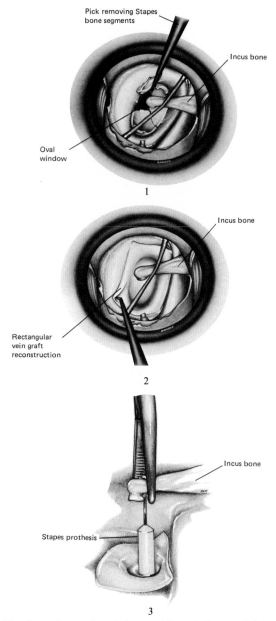

Pick removing Stapes
bone segments

Incus bone

Oval
window

1

Incus bone

Rectangular
vein graft
reconstruction

2

Incus bone

Stapes prothesis

3

Fig. 6-8(a). 1. The diseased stapes bone is fractured from the incus and the oval window and the fragments removed. 2. The oval window is covered with a rectangular vein graft. 3. The wire of the stapes prosthesis is slipped over the incus and closed with forceps. The lower end of the piston is packed to hold it in place during healing. (Courtesy *Richards Mfg. Co. Inc.*)

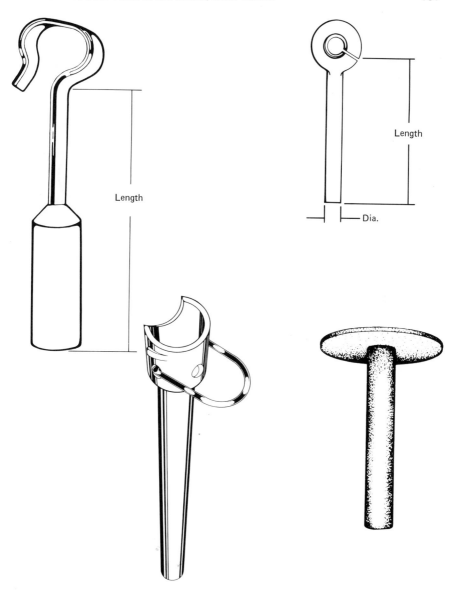

Fig. 6-8(b). Four of the many different designs of ossicular replacement prostheses. 1. Teflon®-platinum ribbon piston type prosthesis, length 3.5 to 5 mm, piston diameter .6 and .8 mm. 2. Snap-on type of Teflon piston prosthesis. 3. Shea locking bail prosthesis in stainless steel or Teflon. 4. Shea Plastipore®* Torp®** prosthesis.

*Plastipore® is a registered trademark of Richards Mfg. Co. Inc. porous high density polyethylene which allows rapid tissue growth into the prosthesis for stabilization.
**Torp® is the registered trademark for the total ossicular replacement prosthesis (drum to window) of the Richards Mfg. Co., Inc.

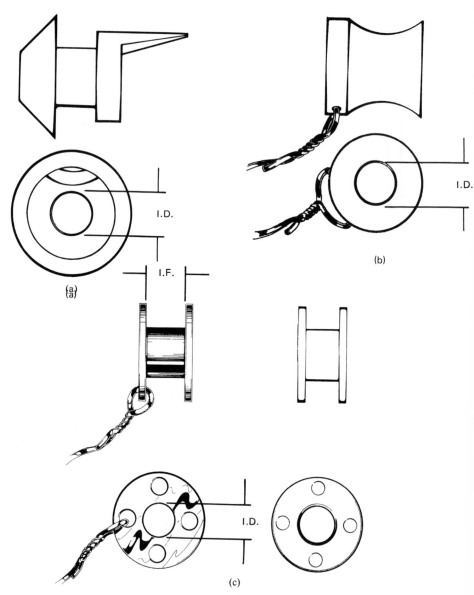

Fig. 6-9. Four of the almost 100 different designs of tympanostomy ventilation tubes. The tabs or wires are to allow forcep removal of the drain. (Courtesy *Richards Mfg. Co., Inc. Memphis, Tenn.*) (a) Shea 'Parasol' silicone drain tube; collapsible flap on left folds during insertion, opens like an umbrella on being placed through the incision (I.D. 1, 1.5 & 2 mm.). (b) Shepard Teflon® grommet drain tube (I.D. 1 & 1.5 mm). (c) Reuter Bobbin stainless steel drain tube (I.D. 1, 1.15 and 1.25 mm). (d) Pope beveled grommet polyethylene drain tube.

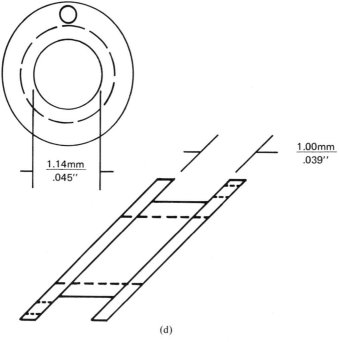

1.14mm
.045''

1.00mm
.039''

(d)

Fig. 6-9. (Continued)

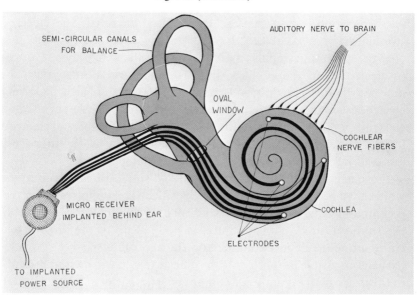

SEMI-CIRCULAR CANALS
FOR BALANCE

AUDITORY NERVE TO BRAIN

OVAL
WINDOW

COCHLEAR
NERVE FIBERS

MICRO RECEIVER
IMPLANTED BEHIND EAR

COCHLEA

ELECTRODES

TO IMPLANTED
POWER SOURCE

Fig. 6-10. Inner ear illustrating cochlear implant. Sound waves entering the ear are normally transmitted via the oval window through the spiraled cochlea, where they stimulate nerve fibers that signal the brain. In the sensory deaf individual, some hearing may be restored by the electrical stimulation of electrodes positioned at selected points along the cochlea.

139

reaches its maximum amplitude closest to the oval window when responding to high frequencies; as the frequency is lowered, the maximum amplitude is reached at increasing distances from the oval window. Thus the frequency of a sound appears to be distinguished by the location of the maximum amplitude of the traveling wave along the basilar membrane. A low volume sound will activate a small number of nerve fibers. As the sound is increased in loudness, apparently more and more nerve fibers adjacent to the point of maximum amplitude are brought into play, signaling to the brain the degree of loudness as well as the pitch of the sound.

Damage to the cochlear hair cells resulting from disease or ototoxic drugs can lead to total, irreversible deafness. The possibility of restoring a degree of hearing by electrical neurostimulation has been pursued for many years; however, it is only in the last decade that some clinical investigations of intracochlear electrical stimulation have shown the promise of near future success for an implantable cochlear prosthesis.[11,12]

Eddington,[13] Dobelle, and Mladejovski at the University of Utah have been applying electrical stimulation through electrodes located at selected points along the cochlea. When activated, the electrodes stimulate the nerves directly with tiny electric shocks which are conveyed as sound signals to the brain. Initially, with only one or a pair of electrodes in the cochlea, only rudimentary sounds such as an automobile horn or doorbell could be recognized. With six or eight electrodes some simple words can be understood. Refinements in the electrode system will eventually allow very large numbers of electrodes in the limited space of the cochlea. This will naturally improve the range of intelligible speech for the deaf patient.

Presently, stimulation is supplied by standard sized computers which have been programmed to deliver electrical impulses to electrode combinations that will originate auditory nerve signals most resembling the sound desired. The computer is hooked up to the implant via a transcutaneous electrical connector, the outer shell of which is made of tissue-compatible pyrolitic carbon. The next step will include reduction of the microphone-computer component to a battery powered unit, the size of a heart pacemaker which will relay its signals to the electrode array via an RF induction coil implanted under the skin.[14] This would be a prosthesis, and its development is quite possible.

VOICE RESTORATION AFTER LARYNGECTOMY

Anatomy of the Larynx

Voice production occurs in the larynx, a box-like structure located between the upper trachea and the base of the tongue. Man has an unusually well-developed larynx which makes possible his sophisticated speech capabilities. The larynx supports the vocal cords. During breathing, the vocal cords are separated. When speech begins, the cartilages of the larynx are drawn together by the action of the muscles and a reed situation is created. (Fig. 6-11). The degree of tension on the vocal cords, which is controlled by the position of the cartilages, alters the pitch of the spoken sound; high notes being produced by the vibration of tight cords, low notes by more relaxed cords.

Cancer is the most common etiology necessitating total laryngectomy. Following surgical removal of the larynx, a prime consideration,

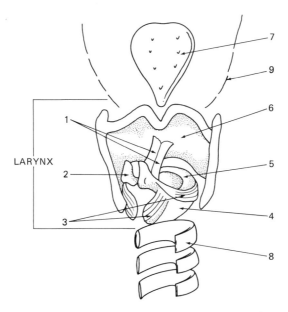

Fig. 6-11. Posterior view of the cartilages of the larynx. 1. Vocal cords under tension are attached in front to the mid-point of the thyroid cartilage, in the back to the arytenoid cartilages. 2. The arytenoid cartilages. 3. The laryngeal muscles which, through manipulation of the arytenoid cartilages control the position of the vocal cords. 4. The crycoid cartilage. 5. Anterior section of the crycoid cartilage—adam's apple. 6. Thyroid cartilage. 7. Laryngeal surface of epiglottis. 8. Tracheal rings. 9. Base of tongue.

naturally, is restoration of the voice. During the last century, a number of artificial larynxes have been designed and tried with very low acceptance. Esophageal speech, in which air swallowed into the stomach is forcibly expelled through the esophagus, is probably the most common means of rehabilitation today. Unfortunately, a high percentage of laryngectomy patients are unsuccessful at developing this type of speech. Several methods of surgical reconstruction of a pseudoglottis have been reported during the past 15 years with varying degrees of success.[15-21] The main difficulty has been the inability of the patient to tolerate them. Postoperative care of a reconstructed pseudoglottis is difficult as are the new swallowing techniques which must be learned. The major problem which contraindicates this type of surgery, since radiation therapy is popularly used to control the spread of cancerous tissue, involves the dehiscence of the irradiated tissue.

In 1969, Dr. Mario Staffieri of Piacenza, Italy pioneered a surgical procedure* in which a flap of esophageal wall was used to close the top of the trachea. A small slit made in the esophageal wall, acts as a valve linking the trachea and the pharynx. To speak, the patient places a finger over the tracheal stoma, this forces air expelled from the lungs to be shunted through the slit valve, thereby allowing phonation. Although the voice is on the raspy side, it is (shortly after surgery) of considerably better quality than that produced by other methods.

Dr. George A. Sisson,† after observing the Staffieri technique and results, tried this approach in the United States but soon discovered that despite apparent initial success in achieving a good voice, serious complications such as aspiration and stenosis of the shunt can occur. It appeared to Sisson and others‡ that the use of a prosthetic valve placed into the shunt opening would be required. Such a valve would stop saliva and food from entering the trachea from the esophagus and thus prevent choking. Ideally the design of the prosthesis should allow easy customization in order to accommodate the local anatomical variations of each patient.

A surgical-prosthetic method for post-laryngectomy speech rehabilitation is illustrated in Figures 6-12 a to d and 6-13. In Fig. 6-12 a

---

*TIME, June 25, 1979.
†George A. Sisson, M.D. Professor and Chairman, Department of Otolaryngology and Maxillofacial Surgery, Northwestern University.
‡Mark I. Singer M.D., Indianapolis, Indiana.[22] William R. Panje, M.D., Department of Otolaryngology and Maxillofacial Surgery, University of Iowa Hospitals, Iowa City, IA 52242[23]

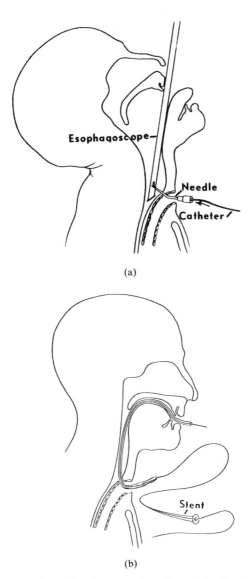

(a)

(b)

Fig. 6-12. (a) The tracheal-esophageal puncture is performed. (b) The Northwestern Surgical Stent is introduced. (c) The stent has dilated the tracheal-esophageal puncture to size. Healing will take place around the silicone rubber without the tissue adhering to it. (d) The Ossof-Sisson laryngectomy tube is in place securing the stent.

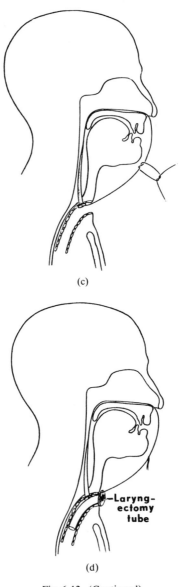

(c)

(d)

Fig. 6-12. (Continued)

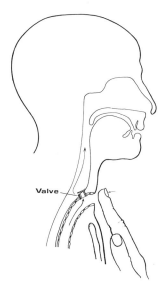

Fig. 6-13. The prosthetic voice restoration valve has replaced the stent in the tracheal-esophageal fistula.

fiber-optic esophagoscope with a perforation in the beveled surface is passed through the oral cavity into the hypopharynx. When the perforation in the esophagoscope can be palpated at the tracheal stoma, a 14-gage disposable I.V. catheter set needle is used to make a puncture through the posterior tracheal wall and into the esophagus at the esophagoscope perforation. The I.V. catheter is then passed through the needle up into the esophagoscope. The needle and the esophagoscope are withdrawn. The string of a Northwestern Surgical Stent (a soft, tapered silicone rubber device, 4.5 mm at the maximum diameter, flanged, and molded around a long length of polyester suture, Fig. 6-12b) is passed up the catheter through the oral cavity where traction is applied, pulling the stent into the esophagus until the flange is against the posterior tracheal wall. The string is then drawn from the oral cavity, through the nose, using a rubber catheter. The string from the nose is then tied to the trailing end from the stent. Fig. 6-12c. The loop of stent string is then taped out of the way behind the patient's ear. An Ossoff-Sisson laryngectomy tube is then placed through the tracheal stoma and held with a neck strap (Fig. 6-12d). In about 48 hours the laryngectomy tube and stent can be removed. The stent is then replaced by a prosthetic valve (Fig. 6-13). When the laryngectomee wishes to speak, the tracheal stoma is blocked with a finger. Air from the lungs is then shunted through the valve and the esophagus into the pharynx allowing the person to phonate. The new voice can be sustained about as long as normal speech. It has a raspy quality but is much superior to other methods of voice restoration.

REFERENCES

1. Dobelle, W. H., et al. "Braille" reading by a blind volunteer by visual cortex stimulation. *Nature* **259**(5539):111–112 (1976).
2. Hirschman, H. Advantages and disadvantages of the types of intraocular lens available. *Trans. Am. Acad. Ophthalmol. Otol.* **81**:89–92 (1976).
3. Kelman, C. D. Phaco-emulsification and aspiration. *Am. J. Ophthalmol.* **67**(4):464–477 (1969).
4. Jaffe, N. S. The changing scene of intraocular implant lens surgery. *Am. J. Opthalmol.* **88**(5):819–828 (1979).
5. Bellucci, R. J. Trends and profiles in stapes surgery. *Ann. Otol. Rhinol. Laryngol.* **88**(5):708–713 1979.
6. Shea, J. J. A 20 year report on fenestration of the oval window. *Trans. Am. Acad. Ophthalmol. Otolaryngol.* **82**:21–29 (1976).
7. Shea, J. J. The use of Proplast™ in otological surgery. *The Laryngoscope* **84**(10):1835–1845 (1974).
8. Marshak, G., and Ben Neriah, Z. Adenoidectomy vs. tympanostomy. *Ann. Otol. Rhinol. Laryngol. Suppl. 68* **89**(3):316–317 (1980).
9. Goode, R. L. The T-tube for middle ear ventilation. *Arch. Otolaryngol.* **97**:402–403 (1973).
10. von Békésy, G. *Experiments in Hearing.* New York: McGraw-Hill, 1960.
11. Mladejovski, M. G., et al. Artificial hearing for the deaf by cochlear stimulation: pitch modulation and some parametric thresholds. *Trans. Am. Soc. Artif. Int. Organs* **31**:1–6 (1975).
12. Tonndorf, J. Cochlear prostheses. *Ann. otol. Rhinol. Laryngol. Suppl. 44* **86**(6): (1977).
13. Eddington, D. K., et al. Auditory prostheses research with multiple channel intracochlear stimulation in man. *Ann. Otol. Rhinol. Laryngol. Suppl. 53* **87**(6): (1978).
14. Hambrecht, F. T. Current status of multichannel cochlear prostheses. *Ann. Otol.* **88**:729–733 (1979).
15. Goode, R. L. The development of an improved artificial larynx. *Trans. Am. Acad. Ophthalmol. Otolaryngol.* **73**:279–287 (1969).
16. Conley, J. Surgical techniques for the vocal rehabilitation of the postlaryngectomized patient. *Trans. Am. Acad. Ophthalmol. Otolaryngol.* **73**:288–299 (1969).
17. Karlan, M. S. Two-stage Asai laryngectomy utilizing a modified Tucker valve. *Am. J. Surg.* **116**:597–599 (1968).
18. Shedd, D., et al. Reed-fistula method of speech rehabilitation after laryngectomy. *Am. J. Surg.* **124**:510–514 (1972).

19. Asai, R. Laryngoplasty after total laryngectomy. *Arch. Otolaryngol.* **95**:114–119 (1972).
20. Taub, S., and Bergner, L. H. Air bypass voice prosthesis for vocal rehabilitation of laryngectomees. *Am. J. Surg.* **125**:748–752 (1973).
21. Sisson, George A., et al. Rehabilitation after laryngectomy with a hypopharyngeal voice prosthesis. *Can. J. Otolaryngol.* **4**(4):588–594 (1975).
22. Singer, M. I. and Blom, E. D. Tracheoesophageal puncture: a surgical prosthetic method for postlaryngectomy speech restoration. Third International Symposium on Plastic & Reconstructive Surgery of the Head & Neck, New Orleans, April 29–May 4, 1979.
23. Panje, W. R. Prosthetic vocal rehabilitation following laryngectomy; The voice button, *Ann. Otol.* **90**:116–120 1981.

7
Implants for Aesthetic Surgery

Beauty has been sought after and appreciated by man since the beginning of reported time. Research has shown that they are often accepted as being more talented than their less fortunate peers.[1-4] Consequently, a growing number of people have opted for plastic surgery for cosmetic improvement of their body. The modern plastic surgeon has a broad array of devices from which to choose, not only to change the appearance of some feature for purely aesthetic reasons, but also to correct the disfiguring effects of congenital malformation, trauma, or disease.

The face is probably the most common target for cosmetic improvement or repair. Illustrated in Fig. 7-1 are a group of commonly used facial implants. If a certain condition cannot be improved with one of the standard implants, blocks of silicone rubber in varying degrees of softness or Proplast are available. They can be carved to the desired size and shape by the surgeon. The pre- and postoperative results of chin augmentation may be seen in Fig. 7-2. Maxillary augmention combined with a nasal strut is shown in Fig. 7-3. The psychological lift experienced by the patient, which usually accompanies such an improvement, is well worth the effort. Cranial defects may be repaired with custom-made silicone rubber or methyl methacrylate inserts. Although silicone fluids are not allowed for general use by the U.S. Food and Drug Administration because of poor results in the case of breast augmentation, resulting from migration of the silicone and its tendency to cause the formation of lumpy granulation tissue, they are being researched clinically with FDA approval for the treatment of extreme facial deformities. In such cases, subdermal injections of silicone fluid are made over a period of

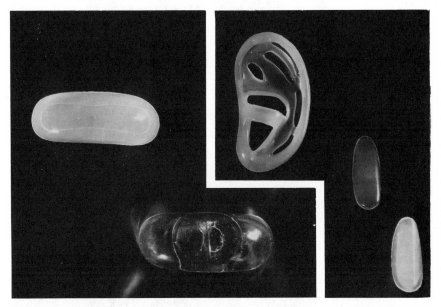

Fig. 7-1. A group of implants for facial reconstruction. *center*: Ear frame around which the plastic surgeon constructs a skin flap contoured to match the natural ear. *left*: Two types of chin implants—one solid, the other softer, gel filled. *right*: Two nose implants for augmentation of "saddle" nose. The whiter of the two has Dacron felt backing to allow tissue ingrowth for attachement. All implants illustrated are manufactured from biocompatible, tissue-like silicone rubber. (*Courtesy of Medical Engineering Corp., Racine, WI 53404*)

time until voids are filled out. A specially treated depeptized collagen[5,6] has also shown promise in clinical trials for the removal by injection of deep wrinkles and pock marks. Figure 7-4 illustrates the use of an implant to effectively correct facial palsy.

In order to achieve a more aesthetically appealing figure, hundreds of thousands of women* with underdeveloped or unevenly developed breasts have undergone breast augmentation with the implantation of a mammary prosthesis. The most popular type of mammary implant consists of a strong, thin, stretchy, transparent silicone rubber shell or sac filled with a clear silicone gel of the same general weight and texture as breast tissue (Fig. 7-5). First developed by Dr. Thomas Cronin of Baylor University, Houston, Texas, these silicone implants are available for breast augmentation and reconstruction in a variety of forms and sizes, allowing the surgeon a broad choice in order to achieve an

*Estimated at over 70,000 per year and growing.

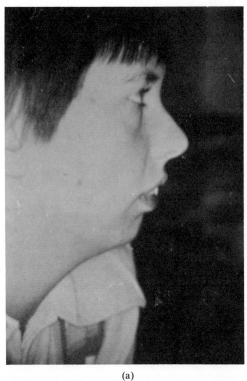

(a)

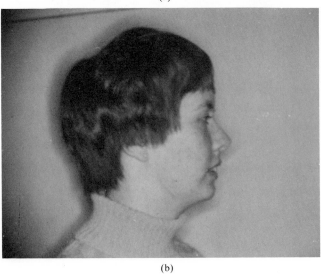

(b)

Fig. 7-2. (a) Preoperative and (b) postoperative profile views of a young woman. The surgeon has performed a mandibular osteotomy, coupled with the implantation of a gel filled chin prosthesis. (*Courtesy of Vaughn Demergian, M.D., Jackson Clinic, Madison, WI 53703*)

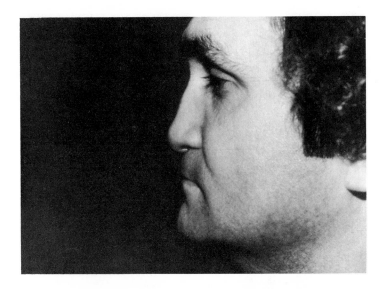

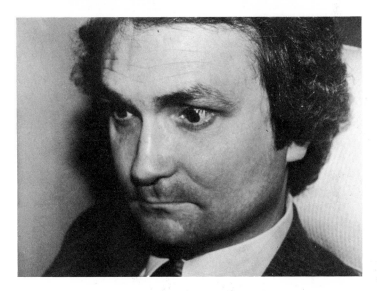

Fig. 7-3. Maxillary augmentation combined with a nasal strut has produced a markedly improved appearance. The implant material used was Proplast. (*Courtesy of Vaughn Demergian, M.D., Jackson Clinic, Madison, WI 53703*)

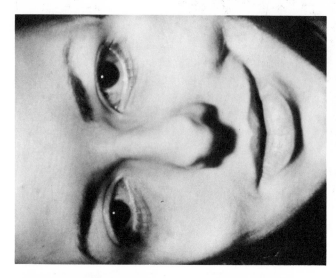

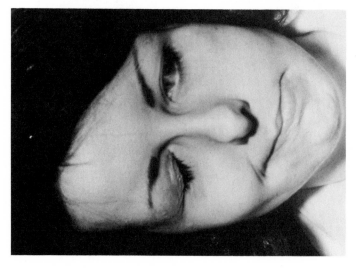

Fig 7-4. Correction of facial palsy utilizing implanted silicone rubber sheeting in place of fascia lata. When synthetic material is used, the trauma of removing the fascia from the thigh is avoided. (*Courtesy of Vaughn Demergian, M.D., Jackson Clinic, Madison, WI 53703*)

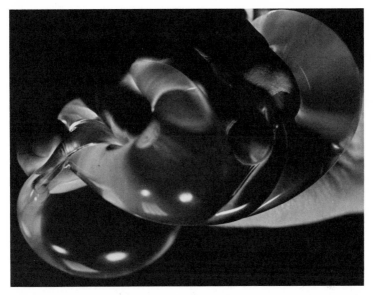

Fig. 7-5. A Surgitek gel filled mammary implant is squeezed strenuously. The photo illustrates the soft, stretchy nature of the silicone materials, combined with their toughness and clarity. Their resistance to high temperatures allows for quick, simple steam sterilization techniques. (*From Handbook of Silicone Rubber Fabrication, Van Nostrand Reinhold, N.Y.*)

optimum comsetic result. A complete list of the profiles and sizes offered by one manufacturer can be found in Table 7-1.

The surgical techniques for inserting the implant under the breast tissue are relatively simple and are often performed under local anesthetic, as an office procedure, requiring on the average no more than one-half hour of actual surgery. There are three surgical techniques used for augmentation mammoplasty; the locations of the incisions are shown in Fig. 7-6.

In the oldest and most common technique, a 4–5 cm incision is made midpoint just above the inframammary fold (Fig. 7-6). The incision is stretched open with retractors and a pocket for the implant is created under the breast tissue by blunt dissection, usually with the surgeon's fingers. After flushing the pocket with sterile saline and antibiotics, and checking to see that all bleeding has been stopped, the surgeon places a sterile implant in the cavity and closes the incision. It is important that the pocket be larger than needed to just accommodate the implant. As is the case with all implants, cells called fibroblasts form a fibrous tissue

Table 7-1. A sample of the Great Variety of Breast Implants Available in Stock Items.*

Low Profile Round Gel-Filled

Volume* (cc's)	(A) Base Diameter (cm's)	(B) Reclining Projection (cm's)
70	8.0	1.5
90	8.5	2.1
110	9.5	2.2
130	10.0	2.3
150	10.5	2.3
170	11.0	2.3
190	11.5	2.3
205	12.0	2.3
220	12.2	2.4
235	12.5	2.4
255	13.0	2.4
270	13.3	2.5
285	13.5	2.5
300	13.7	2.5
320	14.0	2.6
340	14.5	2.7
365	15.0	2.7
400	15.3	2.8
440	15.6	2.8
485	16.0	2.9
600	18.0	3.2

G.B. Snyder Modified Teardrop Gel-Filled

Volume* (cc's)	(A) Base Diameter (cm's)	(B) Projection (cm's)	(C) Height (cm's)
130	8.5	4.7	9.5
165	9.0	4.9	10.0
180	9.5	5.0	10.5
200	10.0	5.1	11.0
235	10.5	5.5	12.0
255	11.0	5.7	12.5
280	11.3	5.9	12.8
300	11.5	6.0	13.0
330	12.0	6.2	13.5
365	12.5	6.4	14.0
400	13.0	6.6	14.5
500	15.5	7.5	17.0

Low Profile Oval Gel-Filled

Volume* (cc's)	(A) Base Diameter (cm's)	(B) Projection (cm's)	(C) Height (cm's)
150	9.5	3.3	11.0
180	10.0	3.5	12.0
210	10.3	3.6	12.5
225	10.6	3.7	13.0
245	10.8	3.7	13.2
265	11.0	3.8	13.5
285	11.5	3.9	14.0
310	11.8	4.0	14.5
350	12.4	4.1	15.0

*Courtesy of Medical Engineering Corp., Racine, WI.

Table 7-1. (Continued)

Oval Gel-Filled

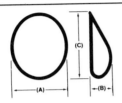

200	10.0	3.2	11.2
215	10.5	3.4	11.6
235	11.3	3.5	12.2
255	11.7	3.6	12.5

Contour Georgiade Gel-Filled

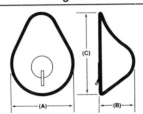

100	8.2	4.5	10.1
140	9.1	4.6	11.4
165	9.5	4.8	11.7
185	10.0	5.4	12.2
225	10.8	6.1	12.8
265	11.0	6.5	13.0
300	13.5	6.6	13.1
360	14.5	6.7	13.2

High Volume Bi-Lumen

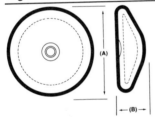

Size (cc's)	Inner Gel (cc's)	Minimum Amount of Saline to be added (total fill cc's)	Maximum Amount of Saline to be added (total fill cc's)	(A) Base Size at Maximum Fill (cm's)	(B) Projection (cm's)	(C) Height (cm's)
70/135	70	40(110)	65(135)	8.4	3.5	
130/210	130	40(170)	80(210)	10.0	3.8	
170/270	170	40(210)	100(270)	10.7	4.3	
205/315	205	50(255)	110(315)	11.8	4.5	
255/375	255	50(305)	120(375)	12.3	4.5	
300/450	300	70(370)	150(450)	13.6	4.5	
340/500	340	70(410)	160(500)	13.8	4.5	
400/600	400	90(490)	200(600)	15.2	4.6	

Low Volume Bi-Lumen

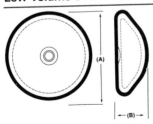

110/140	110	20(130)	30(140)	9.1	3.5
130/160	130	20(150)	30(160)	9.7	3.6
150/180	150	20(170)	30(180)	10.4	3.7
170/205	170	20(190)	35(205)	10.7	3.8
190/230	190	25(215)	40(230)	11.1	4.0
205/250	205	30(235)	45(250)	11.6	4.3
220/265	220	30(250)	45(265)	11.8	4.3
235/285	235	35(270)	50(285)	12.1	4.4
255/310	255	35(290)	55(310)	12.5	4.5
285/345	285	40(325)	60(345)	13.3	4.5
320/385	320	45(365)	65(385)	13.8	4.5
365/435	365	50(415)	70(435)	14.7	4.5
440/520	440	60(500)	80(520)	15.2	4.6

Table 7-1. (Continued)

Contour Georgiade Bi-Lumen

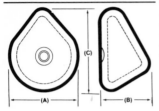

140/165	140	20(160)	40(180)	9.8	3.5	11.4
165/185	165	25(190)	50(215)	10.1	4.0	12.1
185/225	185	40(225)	60(245)	10.4	4.5	12.3
225/265	225	40(265)	70(295)	11.0	5.0	13.0
265/300	265	40(305)	80(345)	13.4	5.4	13.0
300/360	300	60(360)	100(400)	14.4	5.8	13.0

Gel/Saline

Size Delivered Volume (cc's)	Recommended* Amount of Saline to be added (total fill cc's)	Maximum Amount of Saline to be added (total fill cc's)	(A) Base Size at Maximum Fill (cm's)	(B) Projection (cm's)
70	20(90)	50(120)	9.3	2.3
90	30(120)	60(150)	9.8	2.3
110	30(140)	70(180)	10.5	2.4
130	40(170)	80(210)	11.0	2.8
150	40(190)	90(240)	12.0	2.9
175	50(225)	100(275)	12.5	2.9
200	50(250)	120(320)	13.0	3.0
230	60(290)	140(370)	14.6	3.0
270	60(330)	160(430)	15.0	3.1
325	70(395)	170(495)	15.0	3.3
400	80(480)	180(580)	15.5	3.3

capsule around the implant. A special type of fibroblast called a myofibroblast[7,8] can cause the capsule to contract and constrict the implant, which produces a relatively hard and unnatural looking breast profile. This effect may be minimized through the use of a large pocket and daily manipulation of the breast about the pocket in order to effect the loosest possible capsule.[9] A number of plastic surgeons also apply steroids to the pocket, with some degree of success, to aid in controlling contraction. Some prescribe a high daily dosage of vitamin E as well.

Another surgical technique involves a circumareolar (or periareolar) incision. The incision follows the lower half circumference of the areolar border (Fig. 7-6). This technique is popular because it is difficult to detect the incision scar after healing. A variation of this procedure is the Pitanguy transareolar incision.[10] Advantages claimed for this procedure include: early manipulation without undue stress on a suture line, less probability of hematoma, no loss of nipple sensibility, and ease of correction of an inverted nipple.

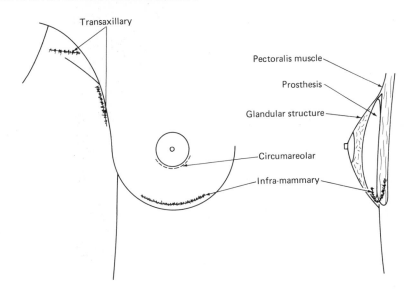

Fig. 7-6. Three locations for incisions in breast augmentation. The prosthesis is shown implanted behind the mammary glandular tissue and in front of the pectoral muscle. There is a growing trend to implant the prosthesis under the muscle,[12–14] especially where a moderate degree of breast enlargement is desired. It is claimed that there is a very low incidence of capsule formation, with a very acceptable long term appearance. (*Adapted from Chirurgie Plastique de Sein, Masson et Cie, Paris, 1974*)

The third surgical approach is referred to as transaxillary; here, the incision is made in the area of the armpit (Fig. 7-6) and consequently the incision scar is completely hidden. Because this method has been accompanied by more complications than the other two, it has not become as popular.

Some surgeons prefer to use a style of mammary implant in which the silicone rubber shell is filled with sterile saline solution instead of a gel. The saline is injected into the shell through a valve at the time of surgery, the shell already having been placed through the incision and into the pocket; these devices are referred to as inflatables. Although the saline is slightly heavier than breast tissue, its advantages over the prefilled gel devices are considered to be: it can easily be inserted through a smaller incision; the volume is adjustable at surgery, which is particularly attractive when there is asymmetry of the breasts; and, finally, the breasts have a livelier feel when palpated. However, there is the probability over a period of time of a small break occuring in the

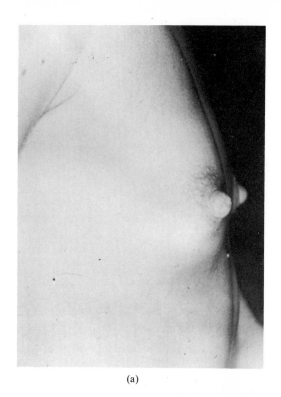

(a)

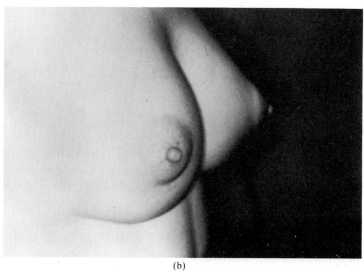

(b)

Fig. 7-7. (a) A preoperative view of the chest of a young woman exhibiting minimal breast development (hypomastia). (b) A postoperative view after augmentation with gel filled implants. (*Courtesy of Vaughn Demergian, M.D., Jackson Clinic, Madison, WI 53703*)

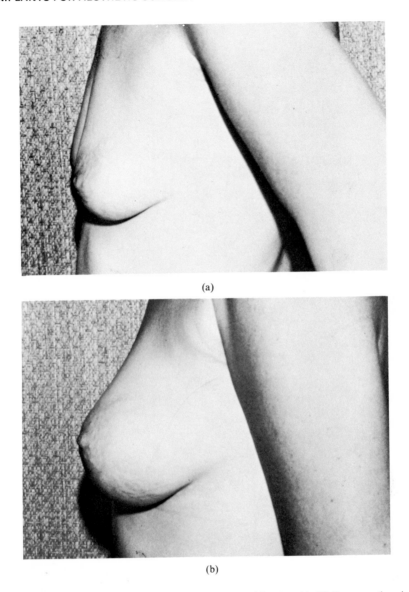

(a)

(b)

Fig. 7-8. (a) Preoperative view of a drooping breast condition (ptosis). (b) Postoperative view illustrating correction with gel filled implants. (*Courtesy of James L. Baker, M.D., Winter Park, FL 32789*)

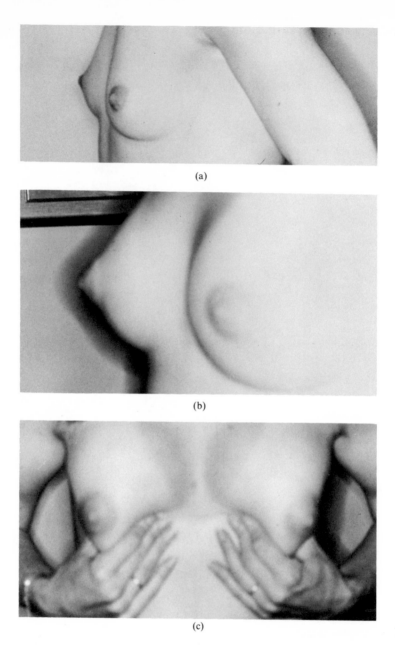

(a)

(b)

(c)

Fig. 7-9. (a) Preoperative view of a young woman whose breast development is not in proportion to the rest of her body. (b) Postoperative view of the same breasts—Surgitek gel/saline implants have been used for augmentation. (c) Demonstration of the natural softness of the breasts 18 months after surgery. (*Courtesy of Vaughn Demergian, M.D., Jackson Clinic, Madison, WI 53703*)

160

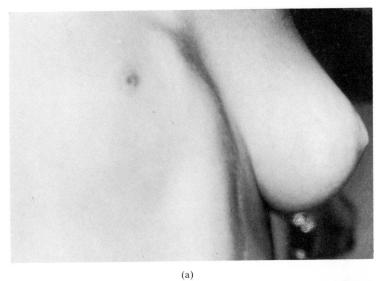

(a)

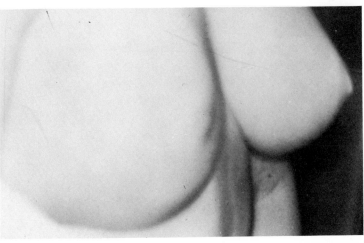

(b)

Fig. 7-11. (a) Preoperative view of a young woman with a chest wall deformity. (b) Postoperative view: a custom-contoured implant has been used to correct the condition. (*Courtesy of Vaughn Demergian, M.D., Jackson Clinic, Madison, WI 53703*)

with simultaneous subcutaneous insertion of a Georgiade Surgitek bi-lumen prosthesis consisting of an inner envelope filled with 165 cc of silicone gel and the outer inflatable envelope filled with 25 cc of saline containing 10 mg of Solu-Medrol. In performing a subcutaneous mastectomy the surgeon removes glandular tissue only, leaving the skin and nipple intact; a silicone prosthesis then replaces the diseased

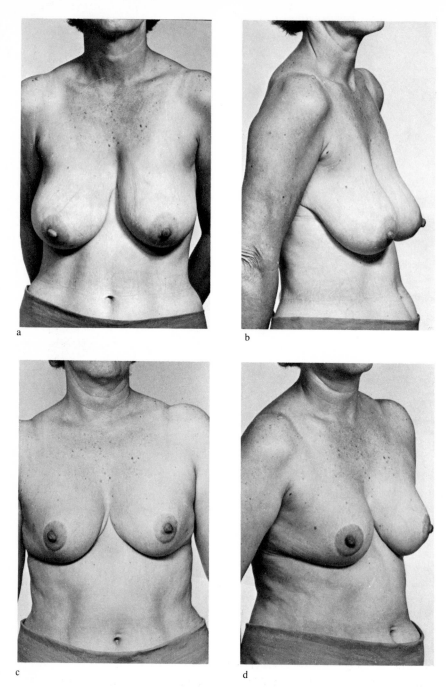

a

b

c

d

Fig. 7-12. (*Courtesy of Nicholas G. Georgiade, M.D., Duke Medical Center, Durham, NC*)

164

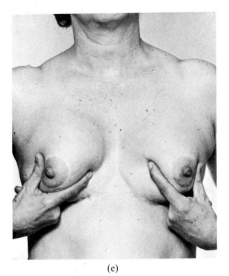

(e)

Fig. 7-12. (Continued)

tissue. Usually performed because of lumpy breast tissue which may become cancerous, this operation is sometimes used prophylactically when family history indicates a high risk of cancer and the individual is highly fearful of the disease. In Fig. 7-12(e), the same 18-month postoperative front view is shown, demonstrating the natural softness of the breasts.

Figures 7-13(a) and (b) show a preoperative front and lateral views of a 53-year-old patient who had a modified radical mastectomy of the left breast. Figures 7-3(c) and (d) present one-year postoperative front and lateral views of the same patient. The left breast has been reconstructed by the insertion of a "piggyback" prosthesis,* consisting of a 100 cc Georgiade Surgitek gel filled prosthesis bonded to a 185 cc

---

*In order to obtain a desired projection without the drooping or flattening of a single large implant, Dr. Georgiade often adheres two devices together and implants them with the smaller of the two in front.

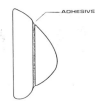

"Piggy Back Prosthesis"

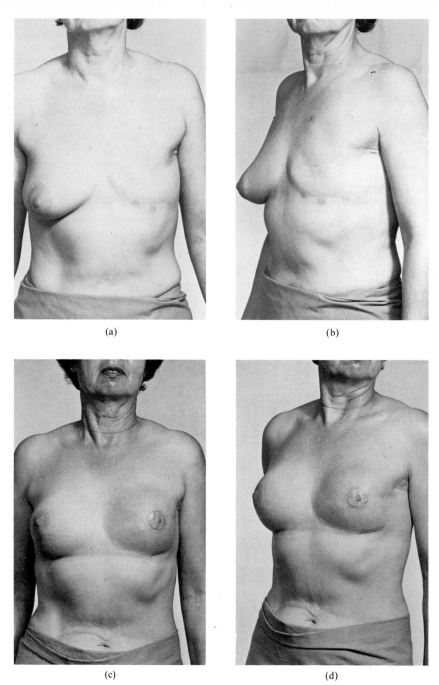

(a)

(b)

(c)

(d)

Fig. 7-13. (*Courtesy of Nicholas G. Georgiade, M.D., Duke Medical Center, Durham, NC*)

Georgiade Surgitek gel filled prosthesis. The nipple-areola complex was reconstructed by nipple-areola sharing from the opposite breast. A subcutaneous mastectomy was performed on the right breast with simultaneous insertion of a 185 cc Georgiade Surgitek gel filled contoured prosthesis. The results obtained are superb.

Successful surgical correction of anomalies or disfiguring trauma can improve self-esteem dramatically. The individual is usually found to have increased confidence and improved overall personal appearance and, as a result, is more relaxed socially.

REFERENCES

1. Landy, D. Beauty is talent. *J. Pers. Soc. Phychol.* **29**:299 (1974).
2. Dion, K., et al. What is beautiful is good. *J. Pers. Soc. Psychol.* **24**:285 (1972).
3. Walster, et al. Importance of physical attraction in dating behaviour. *J. Pers. Soc. Psychol.* **4**:508 (1966).
4. Reich, J. The surgery of appearance. *Med. J.* **2**:5 (1969).
5. Stenzel, K. H., et al. Collagen as a biomaterial. *Am. Rev. Biophys. Bioeng.* **3**:231 (1974).
6. Knapp, T. R., et al. Injectable collagen for soft tissue augmentation. *Plast. Recon. Surg.* **60**(3):398–405 (1977).
7. Gabbiana, G., et al. Pressure of modified fibroblasts in granulation tissue and possible role in wound contraction. *Experimentia* **27**:549 (1971).
8. Montandon, D., et al. The contractile fibroblast; its relevance in plastic surgery. *Plast. Recon. Surg.* **52**:286 (1973).
9. Smahel, V. Effect of expansion exercises on capsular constriction around silicone implants. *Aesth. Plast. Surg.* **3**:339–349 (1979).
10. Pitanguy, I. Transareolar incision for augmentation mammaplasty. *Aesth. Plast. Surg.* **2**(4):363–372 (1978).
11. Rubin, L. R. The deflating saline implant—facing up to complications. *Plast. Recon. Surg.* (May 1980).
12. Woods, J. E., et al. The case for submuscular implantation of prostheses in reconstructive breast surgery. *Ann. Plast. Surg.* **5**(2):115–122 (1980).
13. Pickrell, K. L., et al. Subpectoral augmentation mammaplasty. *Plast. Recon. Surg.* **60**(3):325–336 (1977).
14. Regnault, P. Partially submuscular breast augmentation. *Plast. Recon. Surg.* **59**(1):72–76. (1977).
15. Georgiade, N. G. Breast Reconstruction After Mastectomy. C. V. Mosby & Co. St. Louis, Mo. 1979.

8
Neurological Implants

THE BRAIN, THE NERVOUS SYSTEM AND ELECTRONEURAL STIMULATION

Man's brain is his most remarkable organ. Unlike other organs, which can be explained in terms of familiar equipment (e.g., the heart as a pump, the eye as a camera, the ear as a microphone, etc.), the complex way the brain works is difficult to comprehend. The brain, along with the spinal cord, has sometimes been described as a super computer. Actually, no known computer system can compare with the central nervous system which, although packed in a very small space and using very little energy in comparison to an electronic computer,* can process a tremendous quantity and variety of data as well as being capable of abstract thought.

The brain is made up of nerve tissue which extends down the spinal cord and then, like the wiring harness of a piece of complex electronic equipment, has 31 pairs of separate branches which leave the cord through openings in each vertebra and spread through the body as a fine network of nerves. Figure 8-1 shows the approximate location of the localized centers of the brain having to do with hearing, speech, and vision. The nerve branches from the spinal cord are identified as C (cervical)—8 pairs, T (thoracic)—12 pairs, L (lumbar)—5 pairs, and S (sacral)—5 pairs. The cone-like tapered end of the spinal cord beginning in the upper lumbar region is known as the conus medullaris. A slender thread-like prolongation from the tip of the conus, known as the filum terminale, anchors the spinal cord to the coccyx. The cerebellum located at the base of the skull is that part of the brain which coordinates muscle activity; it does not produce movement but aids in controlling it. Electrical stimulation of the cerebellum has produced

---

*However, the brain takes more of the cardiac output than any other organ—about 25%.

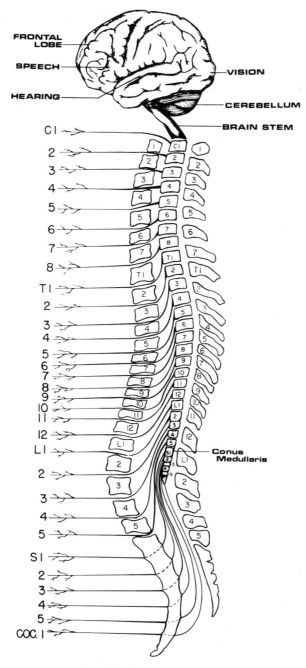

Fig. 8-1. Central nervous system.

relief in cases of spasticity and epilepsy. Stimulation of the central gray matter of the brain, spinal cord, or peripheral nerves has been effective in reducing or eliminating intractable pain in many cases, and stimulation of the conus medullaris has been used with some success in bladder control.

The individual cells of the nerve tissue are known as neurons. The neurons differ in size, and some have specialized functions; however, they all have the ability to transmit the signals that report and control body activities via electrochemical impulses which pass through their tentacle-shaped appendages called axons. Unlike the ordinary electric current traveling in a wire, the electrochemical impulse travels along a nerve fiber without any loss of strength.

The senses such as vision, hearing, smell, and taste communicate directly to the brain. However, many of the nerves connected to the spinal cord are linked only indirectly to the brain; the reaction decision to a signal from them is made at the spinal cord level. For example, if the hand touches a hot object, the receptors in the skin cause an impulse to travel to the spinal cord which in turn sends an impulse to the muscles of the arm, causing a multilevel reflex action, and the hand is jerked away from the heat source. A fraction of a second later, the brain receives the message that the object is hot.

The artificial stimulation of selected nerve tissue by the application of an electric current in order to overcome pain goes back to ancient times when the electric catfish of the Nile (*Malapterurus*) were held to the side of the head to treat headaches. Acupuncture, which is mechanical, probably produces an electrical phenomenon resulting from the twirling of the needles in the nerve tissue; it has been made more effective by some acupuncturists through the application of an electrical current to the needles.

During the 1970s, electronic neurostimulation was widely applied, not only for the successful control of chronic pain in some patients but for an increasing number of clinical problems such as uncontrolled bladder in the paraplegic patient, impaired peripheral vascular circulation, chronic respiratory insufficiency, drop foot, cerebral palsy, multiple sclerosis, epilepsy, dystonia, and others. There is even the potential for crude restoration of sight through visual cortex stimulation and hearing through cochlear nerve stimulation (see Chapter 6).

Pain Relief

The torture of intractable pain affects a significantly large section of the population. It can cost the U.S. economy billions of dollars annually because of loss of earnings, treatment costs, and the not-uncommon abuse of medication and alcohol. Electrotherapy for the treatment of headache and many other conditions had its promoters at various periods of history beginning more than 2000 years ago. For the most part, electrotherapy had been applied very unscientifically and opportunistically by numerous charlatans. Consequently, with the development of modern medical treatment, it fell into disrepute. The successful advent of cardiac pacing, however, helped restore serious interest by the medical community, and today many types of debilitating pain are being relieved by the application of a few coulombs of electricity.

There are a number of transcutaneous electrical nerve stimulation (TENS) devices* on the market. These are devices having electrodes which are placed externally on the surface of the skin. The stimulator delivers a constant pulsed current via the electrodes to the nervous system through nerve endings and nerve trunks located close to the surface of the skin. There are no set rules about the location of the electrodes, and many patients are relieved only after a thorough trial of various locations and stimulation settings. Stimulation current can be set over a range of 0 to 75 mA. The pulse rate varies from 3 to 200 pulses per second. The pulse width may or may not be varied. TENS systems can help manage certain types of chronic pain[1-5] such as phantom limb, neck, and low back syndrome, postherpetic neuralgia, peripheral neuropathies, and arthritis. They may also be effective in treating postsurgical pain as well as the acute pain of dislocations and fractures.

Prior to a decision to use an implantable neurostimulation device, a TENS unit should be used to determine whether there is an incompatibility of the patient to electrical stimulation; some people find the mild prickling sensation quite unpleasant and prefer to use other methods of analgesia.

Implantation of a nerve stimulator is indicated when transcutaneous

*Neuromod—Medtronic, Inc., Neuro Division, Minneapolis, MN 55418; Avery TNS—Avery Laboratories, Inc., Farmingdale, NY 11735, Stimtech—Stimulation Technology, Inc. Minneapolis, MN 55428.

stimulation proves to be ineffective, when an excessively wide area of skin surface must be stimulated to obtain effective relief, or when the electrodes cannot be worn conveniently over the effective stimulation site. The types of implantable nerve stimulators include spinal cord stimulators, deep brain stimulators, and peripheral nerve stimulators.

Because of the relatively high power requirements of neurostimulation along with the desirability of external control of stimulation parameters, external radio frequency power source systems have been developed which convey the stimulation pulse through the skin noninvasively. An implanted miniature radio receiver receives RF signals from an external transmitter equipped with a loop antenna which is taped on the skin directly over the receiver. The RF signals are converted by the receiver into electrical impulses which are conveyed through subcutaneous leads to the electrodes in contact with nerve tissue (see Fig. 8-5).

Spinal Cord Stimulation System. *Spinal cord stimulator systems* apply pulsed electrical stimulation to the dorsal aspect of the spinal cord for the management of chronic intractable pain of the trunk and limbs. The system consists of an external stimulation transmitter connected to an antenna having a flattened doughnut shape and a subcutaneous receiver antenna of the same shape connected to the electrodes. The transmitter may be worn on a belt or in a pocket. Its antenna must be located on the skin directly over the receiver antenna, which has been implanted along with the electrodes. The transmitter antenna is usually taped to the skin. RF signals are transmitted through the skin to the receiver which converts them to minute electrical impulses that are applied to the spinal cord. The best results with this type of stimulation have been obtained in the treatment of phantom limb pain and the intractable pain of low back syndrome.[6]

The Pisces* system allows for trial stimulation by the insertion of leads percutaneously through needles into the spinal cord while the patient is under local anesthesia (see Fig. 8-2 and Table 8-1). The patient can then be interrogated by the physician while the electrode positions are varied to locate the best position for maximum effectiveness and comfort. The patient may go through a trial period of several days before a final decision is made to implant the device for long term stimulation. When permanent implantation is desired, the

*Pisces—trademark, Medtronic, Inc., Minneapolis, MN 55440.

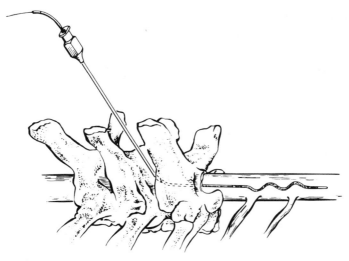

Fig. 8-2. The first electrode is shown placed in the epidural space pointing upward. A second epidural needle will be inserted at the same level or the one below, and an additional electrode and lead will be placed pointing downward. Various parameters of stimulation (amplitude, pulse width, and rate) can then be evaluated. (*Courtesy of Medtronic, Inc.*)

receiver is implanted in a subcutaneous pocket located in the upper chest (similar to a heart pacemaker) or in the abdominal area, and the lead extensions are tunneled subcutaneously and connected to the electrode leads after the temporary lead extensions have been removed. With the RF transmitter and antenna in place, the system is ready for chronic use.

Early in the use of spinal cord (dorsal column) stimulation for intractable back pain on patients with multiple sclerosis, it was found that they also gained improvement in motor control and sensory appreciation.[7-9] Subsequently, the method has been used for rehabil-

Table 8-1. Pisces Component Design and Specifications.

CHARACTERISTIC	PARAMETER (NOMINAL VALUES)
Pulse amplitude	0–10 V, adjustable into a 500-ohm resistive load (with a cm spacing between antenna and receiver)
Pulse rate	1–120 pulses/sec, adjustable
Pulse width	0.1–1.0 msec, adjustable
Transmitter frequency	460 kHz
Transmitter physical parameters	Weight: 150 g (5.3 oz) Size: 10.5 × 7 × 2.4 cm (4.1 × 2.8 × 9 in.)
Battery type	9 V transistor battery

itation of patients with multiple sclerosis in addition to its broader use in pain control. Also noted when the spinal cord was electrically stimulated was the production of regional vasodilation[10] accompanied by increased skin temperature and healing in the case of peripheral vascular disease.

Deep Brain Stimulation System.   Chronic intractable pain of central origin, from facial anesthesia dolorosa to severe post-traumatic pain syndromes involving the spinal cord and peripheral nerves which have been unresponsive to other forms of treatment, has been managed with an encouraging rate of success by electrical brain stimulation.[11-14] The Medtronic DBS* brain stimulation system (Table 8-2) has two basic components: a transmitter-antenna worn externally by the patient, similar to that described for the Pisces system which generates RF pulses, and an implanted receiver-lead, which receives the impulses and sends them to the brain to block the pain signals. The DBS lead is composed of four Teflon insultated platinum wires; at the end proximal to the stimulation target the wires are formed into four electrodes. The proximal electrode is formed into a .9 mm loop. Each electrode is 1 mm long. The distance between the electrodes is 2 mm. The distal end of the lead is terminated by four pin connectors molded into a silicone rubber body. The total length of the lead is 22 cm.

Following implantation of the depth electrode in the internal capsule, sensory thalamus, medial thalamus, or midbrain under local anesthesia, the patient is stimulated with various combinations of electrodes to determine the best combination for pain relief and to

---

*Trademark, Medtronic, Inc., Neuro Division, Minneapolis, MN 55418.

Table 8-2. DBS Brain Stimulation System Specifications.

CHARACTERISTIC	PARAMETER (NOMINAL VALUES)
Pulse amplitude	0–10 V, adjustable into a 500-ohm resistive load
Pulse rate	1–120 pulses/sec, adjustable
Pulse width	.10–1.0 msec, adjustable
Transmitter frequency	460 kHz
Slope rise time	2–30 sec
Current drain	Not to exceed 30 mA
Physical dimensions	10.5 × 7 × 2.4 cm (4.1 × 2.8 × .9 in.)
Weight	212 g (7.5 oz)
Battery type	9 V transistor battery recommended

verify the efficacy of the lead position. When correct placement of the electrodes has been ascertained, a percutaneous lead extension is brought through the scalp and the patient is stimulated percutaneously for a trial period of one week. When the clinical efficacy of the system has been assured, the RF receiver is placed in a subcutaneous pocket in a subclavicular location; a lead extension is then tunneled subcutaneously from the receiver site to the electrode lead, which has been exposed by opening the scalp under general anesthesia and removing the percutaneous extension. Permanent connections are made, all incisions are closed, and the system is ready to function using the portable battery powered transmitter.

Peripheral Nerve Stimulation System. Incorporating the same principle as the two previous systems—an external transmitter and antenna assembly to produce an RF signal which is picked up by an implanted receiver-electrode assembly and converted into pain blocking electric signals to the nerve, the peripheral nerve stimulator differs in that the electrode is a silicone rubber cuff in which four electrodes are embedded (Fig. 8-3). When the cuff is wrapped around the nerve to be stimulated and sutured closed, the electrodes are in contact at four different points on the perineurium. The leads which have color-coded connector pins can then be plugged into transmitter connectors, and stimulation trials to obtain the most efficacious combination can be begun. By exciting the leads in various combinations (e.g., one with each one of the others, pairs with one of the others, different pairs), a total of 21 different paths of stimulation, through the nerve, is possible. Optional conduction paths are essential since individual nerve fiber bundles within the trunk represent

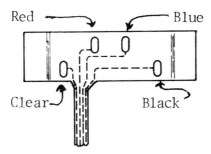

Fig. 8-3. Inside view of nerve cuff layed open. *(Courtesy of Avery Laboratories, Inc., Farmingdale, NY 11735.)*

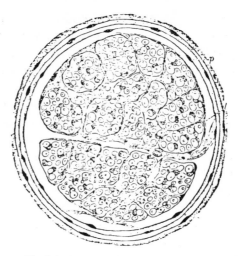

Fig. 8-4. Transverse section through a nerve.

communication lines that monitor or control different functions (Fig. 8-4). The only way to excite the desired nerve sections is by trial and error. The Avery nerve cuffs are available in four sizes: 5, 7.5, 10, and 12 mm.

Upon achieving satisfactory stimulation results, the receiver-antenna unit is implanted in a subcutaneous pocket in a convenient location and the electrode leads which are subcutaneously tunneled to it are connected. The unit is tested, and if it is functioning satisfactorily, the incisions are closed. The system is then ready to operate.

Unfortunately none of the methods described for the management of pain brings complete relief and in many cases there is no relief at all. However, when positive results are obtained, they are dramatic. Stimulation does not have to be applied continuously (e.g., the effect of stimulation for 20 minutes might last for two to three hours initially, but gradually increase up to six or eight hours with no significant pain.[15] There is not the addictive risk of narcotic analgesics or the serious side effects which can occur when conventional neurosurgical lesions are made in an attempt to manage diffused pain.

An Electronic Diaphragm Pacing System

The usual therapy when respiratory paralysis accompanies quadriplegia involves intermittent or permanent use of a mechanical ventilator as well as maintenance of a permanent tracheotomy stoma. Permanent artificial ventilation probably means permanent institutionalization, the risk of recurrent tracheal-pulmonary or systemic infection, and the near impossibility of speech. If the lungs, diaphragm, and phrenic nerves which control the diaphragm are viable, then programmed electrical stimulation of the phrenic nerves can free many cases of respiratory insufficiency from mechanical respiratory support either fully or for a substantial part of the time.[16-18]

In Fig. 8-5, the Yale system of chronic diaphragm pacing developed by Dr. W.W.L. Glenn is illustrated with an Avery Diaphragm Pacemaker. The pacemaker consists of an external RF transmitter with an output signal of 2.04 MH$_2$ which is modulated by a continuous series of pulse trains. Each train of about 35 pulses corresponds to an inspiration period and is adjustable in duration from 1.2 to 1.45 seconds in adults, and 0.5 to 0.8 second in infants. The time interval between one pulse train and the next determines the respiration rate, which is adjustable from 12 to 24 breaths per minute in adults and 12 to 40 breaths in infants.

The *width* of each radiofrequency pulse in the transmitted train determines the *amplitude* of the pulsed current delivered to the phrenic nerve, which in turn controls the depth of the inspiration. During normal operation, the first pulse in the train starts at a relatively small value (about 2.0 mA) and gradually increases until the final pulse (up to

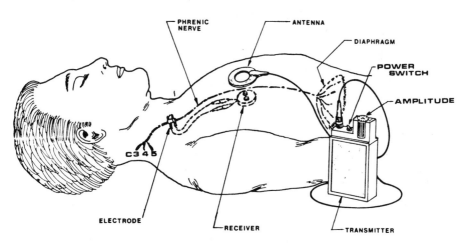

Fig. 8-5. Diaphragm pacer. (*Courtesy of Avery Laboratories, Farmingdale, N.Y. 11735*)

a maximum of 3.0 mA), which determines the maximum extent of the inspiration. This gradual increase provides a near-normal, smooth excursion of the diaphragm as more and more nerve fibers are caused to fire. The graduations can be controlled from very gradual to abrupt. The pulse width of the final RF pulse is controllable so that the maximum current applied to the phrenic nerve can be set at any value up to 10 mA.

The transmitter weighs 227 grams; its dimensions are 73 $\times$ 25 $\times$ 140 mm, and it is powered by a 9 V battery.

A loop antenna consisting of several turns of wire concentrically wound in a flat plane to an outside diameter of 85 mm is connected to the transmitter. It transfers the RF signal from the transmitter to the implanted receiver by inductive coupling through the skin. The antenna is encapsulated with silicone rubber and is usually held in place with hypoallergenic tape.

The receiver contains subminiature integrated electronic circuitry. It contains no batteries, but receives energy and stimulus information from the external antenna by radio waves.

As each radiofrequency (alternating current) pulse in a train is received, it is immediately demodulated, or converted to a direct current pulse of the correct *amplitude* which depends on the pulse *width* of the transmitted signal. The time interval between the beginning of one pulse train and the next (respiration rate) and the length of each pulse train (inspiration time) remain identical to the transmitted signal. The time interval between the end of one pulse train and the beginning of the next allows the diaphragm to relax and is the expiration time.

The demodulated output of the receiver is then capacitively coupled to the electrode, which insures that the net direct current signal applied to the phrenic nerve is electrically zero.

The electronic components of the receiver are hermetically sealed in a metal case, and encircled by a small receiving loop antenna. The entire unit is encapsulated in an epoxy disc and covered with medical grade silicone rubber. This component is 44 mm in diameter and 15 mm thick. It weighs 30.5 grams.

A pair of high strength, highly flexible stainless steel lead wires is attached to the receiver. They are 50 mm in length, coated with medical grade silicone rubber, and are terminated in female stainless steel connectors.

The electrode assembly consists of a silicone rubber cuff in which are embedded two platinum bands having an exposed surface area of 11.5 mm^2. It is designed to be placed around a 1.5 cm segment of mobilized phrenic nerve and to be sutured to the sublying muscle. A pair of high strength, highly flexible stainless steel lead wires, 400 mm long and coated with silicone rubber, connect the electrode to the receiver implant by the use of a pair of pin connectors.

The application of diaphragm pacing is not always successful, but when it is, patients freed from the respirator can participate in many activities including school and gainful employment.

Neurostimulation for the Paralyzed Bladder

Spinal injury leading to paraplegia often interferes with the micturition reflex which controls emptying of the bladder. The use of ureteral catheters either constantly or intermittently, especially at home, can lead to repeated urinary tract infection, kidney malfunction, and consequent shortening of a patient's life. If the conus medullaris (the conical extremity of the spinal cord, see Fig. 8-1) is intact, it is possible by its remote electrical stimulation to control voiding and eliminate the need for catheterization and urine collection devices.[19-24]

The implantation procedure for a micturition stimulator system is similar in principle to that of the peripheral nerve system previously described. The electrode implant* consists of two 2.5 mm insulated platinum electrode pins with 0.5 mm bared tips mounted 2.5 mm apart on an epoxy plastic holder. Two Dacron mesh strips are used to secure the electrode assembly to the conus medullaris after implanting the two electrode pins into the cord (see Fig. 8-6). A RF receiver attached to a Dacron mesh sheet for ease of suturing is placed in a subcutaneous pocket in a flank and connected via a subcutaneous tunnel to the electrodes. The externally carried transmitter generates a pulse modulated RF signal at 2.05 MHz, a frequency selected for lack of interference from outside sources. The pulse width is adjustable from 50 to 400 μsec, the rate from 7 to 200 pulses per second. The amplitude of the transmitter is adjustable. After recovery from surgery (about one week) and the testing of the neuroprosthesis by the physician, the patient is taught to master its use himself. Tensing or spasmodic

---

*As supplied by Avery Laboratories, Inc., Farmingdale, N.Y. 11735

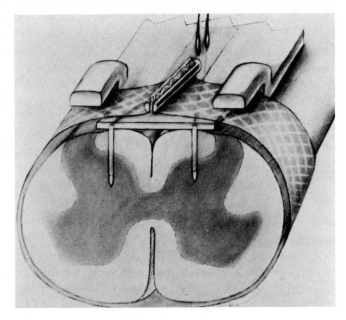

Fig. 8-6. The Avery implant used for electrical stimulation of the conus medullaris in the paraplegic.

movements of the lower extremities are liable to occur during stimulation. However, these become minimal as patients learn to adjust the pulse rate and stimulating voltage for the optimum results. An increase in skin temperature commonly occurs below the spinal lesion while a compensatory cooling takes place above the lesion. Male patients exhibit varying degrees of penile erection with occasional ejaculation. Defecation may also be stimulated, which can be useful in maintaining regularity of bowel movements.

The ability to void at will improves the social confidence of paraplegics and contributes to their being more mobile and independent.

Cerebellar Stimulation for Treatment of Cerebral Palsy and Epilepsy ("The Brain Pacemaker")

The cerebellum (Fig. 8-1) has been associated with certain key motor functions, including the coordination of body muscle activity, equilibrium, and the regulation of muscle tone and posture.[25] The chronic electrical stimulation of the cerebellar cortex seems to cause inhibitory effects on certain neurologic syndromes. Dr. Irving S. Cooper, internationally known pioneer in functional neurosurgery, has reported a statistical study of 50 patients with moderately incapacitating cerebral palsy treated by chronic cerebellar stimulation.[26] Of these patients, 49 showed some beneficial effect varying from marked to mild improvement in speech impairment, spasticity, athetosis, gait impairment, mental functions, self-care, and relaxation. There is a continuing, cumulative improvement of these functions along with a reduction in the stimulation period. Dr. Ross Davis,[27] who has reported on the progress of 75 cerebral palsy patients, points out that cerebellar stimulation reduces spasticity, thereby allowing the other improvements to follow as a result of the patient's residual motor ability. Consequently, if a patient is immature and mentally retarded, he or she will have little motor ability and will only experience the reduction in spasticity. This in itself can be important as far as nursing care is concerned, because in their more relaxed state patients are easier to dress and have improved bowel function. Patients who are mentally alert and have minimal spasticity usually enjoy significant improvement (see Fig. 8-7).

The electrode array differs from others previously described in that it consists of two silicone rubber strips, each of which has four platinum buttons imbedded in a straight line. The silicone pads are soft and flexible with rounded edges to prevent irritation to the surrounding tissue. All eight buttons are now connected to the cathode terminal of a fully implantable constant current pulse generator powered by a lithium-iodine battery (Fig. 8-8). Each platinum button is 8 mm^2 in area, making the total cathodic area 64 mm^2 during any given pulse. The parameters of stimulation for the cerebellar surface are 1 mA and 0.5 msec for the pulse; its rate is 150 pulses per second, with an ON cycle of 4 minutes and an OFF cycle of similar duration. The charge density is 0.8 Coulomb/cm^2/phase which is well below that which causes damage to brain tissue in experiments with monkeys. For pediatric use, the electrode array is approximately one-third smaller than the standard array just described. The implantable pulse generator has been used since May 1979 by Dr. Ross David to replace an external transmitter system similar to that illustrated in Fig. 8-5. Long life lithium-iodine batteries make totally implanted devices possible.

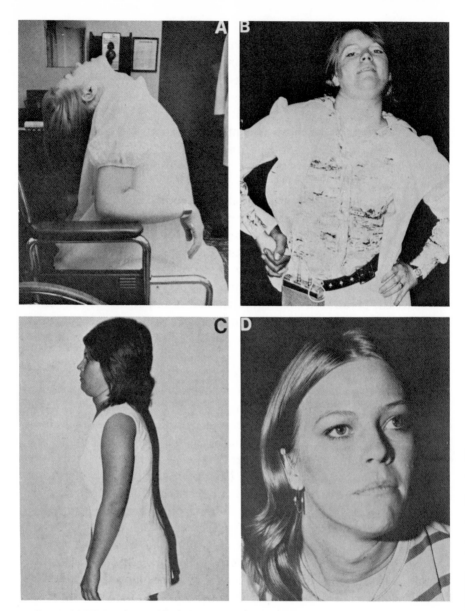

Fig. 8-7. (A) A 20-year-old girl with dystonia suffered severe spine and head retraction (July 1974). (B) Six months following implantation of stimulator on anterior surface of cerebellum. (C) One year after implant. (D) February 1976, (*Courtesy of Dr. Ross Davis, Mt. Sinai Hospital, Miami Beach, FL 33140*)

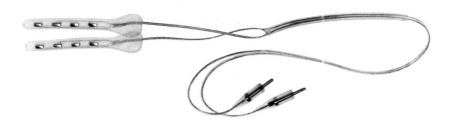

Fig. 8-8. Avery* electrode array used in cerebellar stimulation shown connected to an implantable Neurolith† pulse generator.

During surgery the cerebellum is exposed via two paramedian suboccipital burr holes just 1 cm below and lateral to the occipital protuberance. A subcutaneous pocket is formed for the Neurolith pulse generator in the right abdominal area which is connected via a subcutaneous tunnel to the electrode pads. The two electrode pads are placed, one on each side, anteriorly, between the tentorium and the superior cerebellar surface as shown in Fig. 8-9. The leads are connected, the system tested, and the incisions closed. Since May 1979, 120 patients have had the fully implanted Neurolith pulse generator; no failure of the electronics has yet occurred, and over 90% of the patients report worthwhile reductions (25–50%) of spasticity, allowing them better use of their own limited abilities.[30]

Cooper has also reported the use of chronic cerebellar stimulation in the treatment of 15 patients suffering from intractable, uncontrollable epileptic seizures.[29] Ten of the patients experienced modification or inhibition of their seizures for prolonged periods. They reported being more attentive and alert, and capable of improved work or study activities.

The results of the application of electrostimulation in bone tissue repair, heart and diaphragm pacing, control of pain without depen-

*Avery Laboratories, Inc., Farmingdale, N.Y. 11735
†Neurolith 601—trademark, Pacesetter Systems, Inc., Sylmar, Ca. 91342

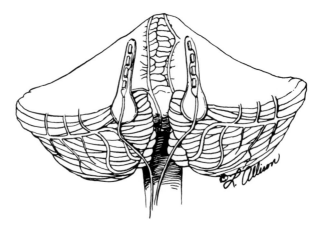

Fig. 8-9. Two electrode pads placed on superior cerebellar surface.

dence on drugs, reduction of spasticity, control of the bladder, and restoration of some degree of hearing are quite remarkable. They encourage a far deeper study of the effects of electricity on biologic systems. The surface has barely been scratched, and with greater knowledge of these phenomena, very specific, nondestructive approaches can be expected in the healing of a multitude of health problems.

A Nonelectronic Implant for the Treatment of Hydrocephalus

Hydrocephalus is a condition characterized by the abnormal accumulation of fluid in the cranial cavity, accompanied by enlargement of the head, particularly the forehead, and atrophy of the brain.

The main source of cerebrospinal fluid is the choroid plexus, fringe-shaped tufts of small capillary vessels situated deep in the ventricles of the brain. The system of the healthy individual absorbs cerebrospinal fluid at the same rate that it is produced. When the absorption system fails to function, fluid pressure builds up in the cranial vaults, compressing brain tissue and enlarging the skull.

Several types of hydrocephalus shunts have been designed to remove excess fluid from the brain and convey it to the heart or peritoneal cavity. This was one of the earliest applications of silicone rubber as an implant material. Hundreds of thousands of children have been kept

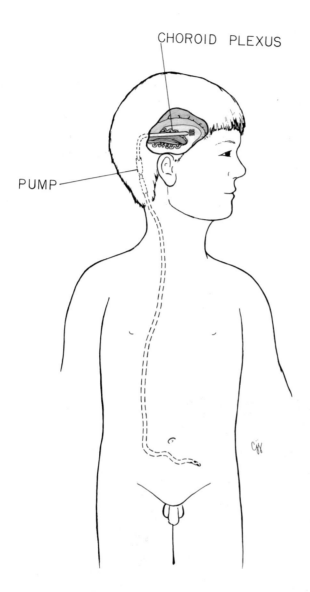

CHOROID PLEXUS

PUMP

Fig. 8-10. Hydrocephalus shunt system: A silicone rubber drainage catheter is placed deep into a ventricle of the brain via a hole drilled through the skull. A right angle bend just external to the skull bone allows a connection to a conduit which has been tunneled under the skin to the abdominal area where another catheter directs the fluid into the perineal cavity. A valve and pumping system is incorporated in the subcutaneous conduit to control the cerebrospinal fluid balance. (The illustration shows a section of skull and brain removed to expose the choroid plexus and indicate the position of the ventricular drainage catheter.)

alive with this system and nave been able to live normal lives. A typical shunt system is illustrated in Fig. 8-10: a silicone rubber drainage catheter is placed deep into a ventricle of the brain via a hole drilled through the skull. A right angle bend just external to the skull bone allows a connection to a conduit which has been tunneled under the skin to the abdominal area where another catheter directs the fluid into the perineal cavity. A valve and pumping system is incorporated into the subcutaneous conduit to control the cerebrospinal fluid balance (Fig. 8-10 shows a section of skull and brain removed to expose the choroid plexus and indicate the position of the ventricular drainage catheter). Figure 8-11 illustrates the catheter for a hydrocephalus shunt. One of the difficulties experienced with drainage catheters has been the blockage of the drain holes in the tip by the delicate fringe-like tufts of the choroid plexus tissue. The silicone rubber catheter tip illustrated in Fig. 8-11 has a series of soft, pliable fins which fold back during insertion (*lower right*). When the catheter is in position, the fins spring back and prevent cellular debris from entering the inlet holes. If the inlet holes become blocked, they may be cleared by applying finger pressure to the subcutaneous pump just behind the ear to produce a back pressure at the holes. This intricate catheter tip is an outstanding example of the precision molding of silicone rubber.

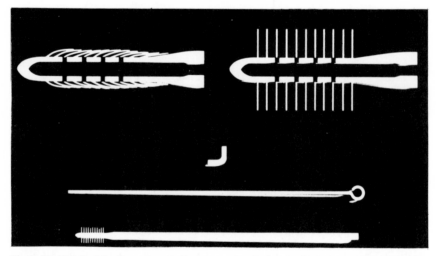

Fig. 8-11. Detail of the tip (enlarged about three times) of a ventricular arainage catheter for hydrocephalus. (*Courtesy of Cordis Corp., Miami, FL; U.S. Patent number 3,516,410*).

Ascites, the effusion into and collection of an excess of serous fluid in the abdominal cavity, can be treated with a similar type of implanted shunt. In this case, the peritoneal catheter drains the abdominal cavity of serous fluid which is pumped through a subcutaneous conduit that carries the fluid via a vein to the heart. In the heart, the fluid is mixed thoroughly with the blood and undesirable constituents are eliminated in the regular waste disposal process.

REFERENCES

1. Andersson, S.A. Pain control by sensory stimulation. *Pain Abstracts* **1**:97 (1978).
2. Burton, C. Transcutaneous electrical nerve stimulation to relieve pain. *Postgraduate Medicine,* **59**(6):105–108 (1976).
3. Loeser, J.D., et al. Relief of pain by transcutaneous stimulation. *J. Neurosurg.* **42**(2):308–314 (1975).
4. Burton, C., and Maurer, D.D. Pain suppression by transcutaneous electronic stimulation. *IEEE Transactions on Biomedical Engineering,* **21**(2):(1974).
5. Nathan, P.W., and Wall, P.D. Treatment of post-herpetic neuralgia by prolonged electric stimulation. *Br M. J.* **3**:645–647 (1974).
6. Burton, C.V. Dorsal column stimulation. *Surg. Neurol.* **4**:171–179 (1975).
7. Cook, A.W., and Weinstein, S.P. Chronic dorsal column stimulation in multiple sclerosis. *NY State J. Med.* **73**(24):2868–72 (1973).
8. Cook, A.W. Electrical stimulation in multiple sclerosis. *Hospital Practice* April 51–58 (1976).
9. Illis, L.S., et al. Dorsal column stimulation in the rehabilitation of patients with multiple sclerosis. *Lancet* 1383–6 (June 26, 1976).
10. Cook, A.W. et al. Vascular disease of extremeties. *N. Y. State J. Med.* **73**(3):366–368 (1976).
11. Mullett, K. Electrical brain stimulation for the control of chronic pain. *Med. Inst.,* **12**(2):88–91 (1978).
12. Richardson, D. E., and Huda, A. Pain reduction by electrical brain stimulation in man. *J. Neurosurg.* **47**:178–194 (1977).
13. Hosobuchi, Y. et al. Chronic thalamic and internal capsular stimulation for the control of facial anesthesia dolorosa and dysesthesia of thalamic syndrome. *Adv. Neurol.* **4**:783–787 (1974).
14. Hosobuchi, Y., et al. Pain relief by electrical stimulation of the central gray matter in humans and its reversal by naloxone. *Science* **197**:183–186 (1977).
15. Richardson, D.E., and Akil, H. Long term results of periventricular gray self-stimulation. *Neurosurgery* **1**(2):199–202 (1977).
16. Glenn, W.W.L., et al. Long-term ventilatory support in quadriplegia. *Ann. Surg.* **183**(5):566–577 (1976).
17. Young, R.F. Diaphragm pacing as an adjunct in respiratory insufficiency. *Neurosurgery* **2**(1):43–46 (1978).
18. Glenn, W.W.L. The treatment of respiratory paralysis by diaphragm pacing. *Ann. Thor. Surg.* **30**(2):106–109 (1980).
19. Boone, E.T. and Self, L.H. Nursing care of the paraplegic using an experimental electronic spinal neuroprosthesis to activate voiding. *J. Neurosurg. Nurs.* **4**:61–74 (1972).

20. Nashold, B.S., Jr., Friedman, H., Glenn J.P., et al. Electromicturition in paraplegia. *Arch. Surg.* **104**:195–202 (1972).
21. Nashold, B.S., Jr., Friedman, H., Grimes, J., and Avery, R. Electromicturition in the paraplegic. *Neural Organization And Its Relevance to Prosthetics.* Miami, Fl. Symposia Specialists 1973, pp. 349–367.
22. Grimes, J.H., et al. Clinical application of electronic bladder stimulation in paraplegics. *J. Urol.* **113**:338–340 (1975).
23. Nashold, B.S., Jr., et al. Operative stimulation of the neurogenic bladder, Neurosurgery Vol. 1, No. 2, 218–220, Sept./Oct. 1977.
24. Letellier, M.A., Moffat, N.A., and Meyer, P.G. Electrical stimulation of the conus medullaris and its effect on the neurogenic bladder. *Wisconsin Med. J.* **77**:S18–S19 (1978).
25. Truex, R., and Carpenter, M. *Strong and Elwyn's Human Neuroanatony,* Sixth Ed., Baltimore, Maryland, Williams and Wilkins, 1969.
26. Cooper, I.S., et al. Chronic cerebellar stimulation in cerebral palsy. Neurology, Minneap. 26:744–753, 1976.
27. Davis, R., et al. Cerebellar stimulation for cerebral palsy. *J. Fl. Med. Assoc.* **63**:910–912 (1976).
28. McLellan, L. et al. Time course of clinical and physiological effects of stimulation of the cerebellar surface in patients with spasticity. *J. Neurol. Neurosurg. Psychiatry* Vol. **41**(2):150–160 (1978).
29. Cooper, I.S., et al. Chronic cerebellar stimulation in epilepsy. *Arch. Neurol.* **33**:559–570 (1976).
30. Davis, R., and Gray, E. Technical problems and advances in the cerebellar-stimulating systems used for the reduction of spasticity and seizures. *Appl. Neurophysiology* (1981).

Glossary

TERMS RELATED TO AESTHETIC AND PLASTIC SURGERY

Alloplasty. Use of a material such as metal or plastic, not from the human body, in plastic surgery.

Aplasia. Lack of development of an organ.

Augmentation mammoplasty. Plastic reconstruction of the breast with an increase of its volume.

Autoplasty. Plastic reconstruction using tissue taken from another part of the patient's body.

Blepharoplasty. Plastic reconstruction of the eyelids.

Capsular contracture. The tough, constrictive, collagenous capsule formed around a foreign body by myofibroblasts.

Genioplasty. Plastic reconstruction of the chin.

Heterograft. Tissue transplant from one species to a different species, e.g., monkey to man.

Homograft. Tissue transplant from one member of a species to another member of the same species.

Hypertrophy. The enlargement or overgrowth of an organ or body part.

Hypomastia. Minimal development of the breasts.

Mastectomy (Mammectomy). Excision of the breast.

Mastopexy. Surgical fixation of a pendulous breast.

Osteotomy. The surgical cutting of a bone.

Otoplasty. Plastic reconstruction of the ear.

Poland's Syndrome. A congenital unilateral defect of the pectoralis muscle (the most common muscle anomaly).

Ptosis. Prolapse of an organ or body part from its normal position.

Reduction mammoplasty. Breast volume reduction by excision of a portion of the gland and skin and usually accompanied by relocation of the nipple.

Rhinoplasty. Plastic reconstruction of the nose.

Rhitidectomy. Surgical removal of wrinkles.

Stroma. The structural elements or framework of an organ.

Subcutaneous mastectomy. A mastectomy in which only the glandular tissue of the breast is removed, leaving the skin and nipple intact.

TERMS RELATED TO THE EAR

Conduction deafness. Deafness due to a defect in the sound conducting parts of the ear.

Myringotomy. Surgical incision of the tympanic membrane.

Otoscleronectomy. Excision of the ankylosed sound conducting bones in the middle ear.

Otosclerosis. The formation of spongy bone in the tympanum causing ankylosis of the sound conducting bones.

Otoscope. An instrument for inspecting the ear.

Pitch. The property of a tone that is determined by the frequency of the sound waves producing it. The quality of the tone is dependent on the number of harmonics present which is why the same pitch sounds different when rendered by different musical instruments.

Sensory deafness. Deafness caused by damage to the cochlear hair cells.

Stapedectomy. Excision of the stapes.

Tinnitis. Varius types of noise occurring in the ears. They may be caused by infection, an involuntary contraction of an internal muscle, a disturbance of the otic nerve, pathological sounds originating from within the body in the region of the ear, or they might be strictly subjective.

Tympanoplasty. Surgical reconstruction of the hearing mechanism of the middle ear with restoration of the drum membrane.

Tympanotomy. Puncture of the tympanic membrane.

Tympanum. The cavity of the middle ear.

TERMS RELATED TO THE EYE

Anterior chamber. Space in the front of the eye, bounded in front by the cornea and behind by the iris; filled with aqueous.

Aphakia. Absence of the lens of the eye.

Aqueous humor. Clear, watery fluid which fills the anterior and posterior chambers within the front part of the eye.

Biconcave lens. Lenses having two concave surfaces on opposite faces.

Bioconvex lens. Lenses having two convex surfaces on opposite faces.

Binocular vision. Ability to use both eyes simultaneously to focus on the same object and to fuse the two images into a single image which gives a correct interpretation of its solidity and its position in space.

Concave lens. Lens having the power to diverge rays of light; also known as diverging, reducing, negative, myopic, or minus lens, denoted by the sign −.

Cones and rods. Two kinds of cells which form a layer of the retina and act as light-receiving media. Cones are concerned with visual acuity and color discrimination; rods, with motion and vision at low degree of illumination (night vision).

Contact lens, corneal. Contact lens for the cornea only.

Contact lens, scleral. Contact lens fitted to the entire globe.

Convex lens. Lens having power to converge rays of light and to bring them to a focus; also known as converging, magnifying, hyperopic, or plus lens, denoted by sign +.

Cornea. Clear, transparent portion of the outer coat of the eyeball forming the front of the aqueous chamber.

Corneal graft. Operation to restore vision by replacing a section of opaque cornea.

Cryosurgery. Use of low temperature in surgery.

Crystalline lens. A transparent, colorless body suspended in the front of the eyeball, between the aqueous and the vitreous, the function of which is to bring the rays of light to a focus in the retina.

- Luxated lens—A condition which occurs when the crystalline lens of the eye is completely displaced from the pupillary aperture.
- Subluxated lens—A condition which occurs when the crystalline lens of the eye is partially displaced but remains in the pupillary aperture.

Cylindrical lens. A segment of a cylinder, the refractive power of which varies in different meridians; used in the correction of astigmatism.

Diopter. Unit of measurement of strength or refractive power of lenses.

Diplopia. The seeing of one object as two.

Discission. Needling of the cateract to permit entrance of aqueous humor and ultimate absorption of lens.

Enucleation. Complete surgical removal of the eyeball.

Erysiphake. Surgical instrument for the removal of a cataractous lens by suction.

Extrinsic muscles. External muscles of the eye which move the eyeball. Each eye has four rectus and two oblique muscles.

Focus. Point to which rays are converged after passing through a lens.

Fovea. Small depression in the retina at the back of the eye; the part of the macula adapted for most acute vision.

Glaucoma. An ocular disease having as its primary characteristic a sustained increase in intraocular pressure which the eye cannot withstand without damage to its structure or impairment of its function.

Hyperopia, hypermetropia. A refractive error in which, because the eyeball is short or the refractive power of the lens is weak, the point of focus for rays of light from distant objects (parallel light rays) falls behind the retina; thus accommodation to increase the refractive power of the lens is necessary for distant as well as near vision.

Hyphema. Hemorrhage in the anterior chamber of the eye.

Intracapsular removal. Removal of the lens with the lens capsule intact.

Intraocular pressure. Pressure of the fluid within the eye.

Iris. Colored, circular membrane suspended behind the cornea and immediately in front of the lens. The iris regulates the amount of light entering the eye by changing the size of the pupil.

Keratectomy. Removal of a portion of the cornea.

Keratoplasty. Corneal graft.

Keratoprosthesis. Corneal implant usually of plastic material; artifical cornea.

Lamellar keratoplasty. Operation in which only diseased outer layers of the cornea are removed and a healthy donor cornea is sutured as a replacement.

Lens:

  Types:

- Aphakic—A convex spectacle lens of high dioptric power, so named because its principal use is in the correction of vision in aphakia.
- Biconcave—A lens with both surfaces concave. Used in myopia ("nearsightedness").
- Biconvex—A lens with both surfaces convex. Used for the treatment of hypermetropia ("farsightedness").
- Bifocal—A lens constructed of two separate lenses each of different power. The upper portion is used for distance vision; the lower portion, for near vision.
- Cross cylinder—A compound lens in which the dioptric powers in the principal meridians are equal but opposite in sign, usually mounted with the handle midway between the principal meridians. Used to determine the axis and the power for correcting astigmatism.

Limbus. Boundary between cornea and sclera.

Macula lutea. Small area of the retina that surrounds the fovea and with the fovea comprises the area of the retina used for distinct vision.

Miosis. Reduction in the size of the pupil.

Mydriasis. Increase in pupil size.

Myopia. "Nearsightedness"—a refractive error in which, because the eyeball is too long in relation to its focusing power, the point of focus for rays of light from distant objects (parallel light rays) is in front of the retina.

Near vision. Ability to perceive objects distinctly at normal reading distance, about 14 inches from the eyes.

Nystagmus. An involuntary oscillating, rapid movement of the eyeball; it may be lateral, vertical, rotary, or mixed.

Optic atrophy. Degeneration of the nerve tissue which carries messages from the retina to the brain.

Optic disc. Head of the optic nerve in the eyeball.

Optic nerve. Special nerve of the sense of sight which carries message from the retina to the brain.

Ora Serrata. Anterior border of the retina.

Orbit. Cavity in the skull which contains the eyeball.

Peripheral vision. Ability to perceive the presence, motion, or color of objects outside of the direct line of vision.

Phacoanaphylaxis. Hypersensitivity to the protein of the crystalline lens.

Posterior chamber. Space between the back of the iris and the front of the lens, filled with aqueous.

Presbyopia. Gradual lessening of the power of accomodation of the near point of distinct vision resulting from the loss of elasticity of the crystalline lens which becomes noticeable at about 40 years of age.

Pupil. Opening at the center of the iris of the eye for the transmission of light.

Rectus muscle. Muscle attached to the eyeball which controls eye movements.

Refraction. (1) Deviation in the course of rays of light in passing from one transparent medium into another of different density. (2) Determination of refractive errors of the eye and correction by glasses.

Refractive error. A defect in the eye that prevents light rays from being brought to a single focus exactly on the retina.

Retina. Innermost tissue layer of the eye, formed of sensitive nerve elements and connected with the optic nerve.

Retinal detachment. Separation of the inner layer of the retina from the outer layer and the choroid.

Schlemm's Canal. Circular channel at the junction of the sclera and cornea through which aqueous humor leaves the eye.

Sclera. White part of the eye—a tough covering which, with the cornea, forms the external, protective coat of the eye.

Scotoma. A blind area of reduced vision in the visual field.

Separation of retina. Separation of the retina from its pigment epithelium layer.

Subluxation of the lens. Incomplete dislocation of the crystalline lens.

Tonography. Determination of the outflow of aqueous humor under the continuous pressure exerted by the weight of a tonometer over a 4- to 5-minute period.

Tonometer. Instrument for measuring the pressure of the eye.

Trephining. Removal of a circular button or disc of tissue.

Uvea. Entire vascular coat of the eyeball. It consists of the iris, ciliary body, and choroid.

Uveitis. Inflammation of the vascular cost of the eye.

Visual acuity. Ability of the eye to perceive the shape of objects in the direct line of vision.

Visual purple. A pigment in the outer layers of the retina; a photochemical substance translating light into nerve impulses.

Vitreous. Transparent, colorless mass of soft, gelatinous material filling the eyeball behind the lens.

TERMS RELATED TO THE HEART AND VASCULAR SYSTEM

Anastomosis. The surgical formation of a passage between two vessels.

Aneurism. A sac formed by the dilation of the walls of a blood vessel.

Arythmia. Absence of a normal heart beat.

Asynchronous pulse generator. A fixed-rate pulse generator in which the rate is independent of the electrical or mechanical activity of the heart.

Atrial synchronous pulse generator. A ventricular pulse generator, the rate of which is determined by the atrial rate.

Auricular tachycardia. Auricular flutter.

Autologous blood. One's own blood.

Basic pulse generator rate. The rate of an implanted pulse generator independent of the electrical or mechanical activity of the heart.

Bradycardia. Slowness of heart beat (60 or less).

Cardioplegia. Interruption of the heart beat which may be induced by chemical compounds or cold in preparation for surgery upon the heart.

Cardiotomy. Surgical incision of the heart.

Diastole. Period of dilation of the heart.

Embolism. Sudden obstruction of a blood vessel by a clot or obstruction such as an air bubble.

Endocardial. Within the heart.

Epicardium. Layer of pericardium which is in contact with the heart.

Escape interval of pacemaker. The time between the sensing of a spontaneous heartbeat and the succeeding output pulse of a triggered pulse generator.

Heart block. Loss of synchronization between the atrial and ventricular muscles. Leads to low heart output (Stokes-Adams disease).

Hemolysis. Separation of the hemoglobin from the corpuscles and its appearance in the fluid in which the corpuscles are suspended.

Homologous blood. Blood from another person.

Hypertension. High blood pressure.

Hypothermia. Induced low body temperature to decrease metabolism of tissues and thereby need for oxygen during certain surgical procedures.

Infarct. An area of necrosis in tissue due to obstruction of circulation to the area.

Ischemia. Deficiency of blood in a part due to constriction or obstruction of a blood vessel.

Myocardium. The middle and thickest layer of the heart wall composed of cardiac muscle.

Nodal bradycardia. Venous tracing show no wave due to contraction of atrium.

Pacemaker (heart pacer). Complete unit of pulse generator, leads and electrodes.

Pericardium. The tough fibrous sac surrounding the heart.

Pulse generator. Part of the pacemaker system that produces a periodic electric pulse.

Pulse interval. Time between the leading edges of successive pulses.

Purse string suture. A continuous running suture placed around an opening and then drawn tight.

Refractory period of pacemaker. The period during which a triggered pulse generator is unresponsive to the input signal.

Stimulation threshold of pacemaker. Lowest amount of energy, measured on the way down, that will consistently pace the heart.

Stasis. Stoppage of the flow of blood.

Systole. Period of contraction of the heart.

Tachycardia. Excessive heartbeat (above 100)

Thromboembolism. Obstruction of a blood vessel which has broken loose from the site of formation.

Thrombogenic. Producing a clot.

Triggered pulse generator. Rate is modified by the electrical or mechanical activity of the heart.

Ventricular fibrillation. Fibrillary twitching of the ventricular muscle, so rapid that coordinated contractions cannot occur.

Ventricular inhibited pulse generator. Delivers a pulse to the ventricle synchronously with the natural ventricular activity. In the absence of ventricular activity it reverts to its basic rate.

TERMS RELATED TO NEUROLOGICAL DEVICES

Athetosis. Involuntary slow, writing movements, especially in the hands.

Autonomic. Self-controlling; functionally independent.

Brainstem. That part lying between the brain and spinal cord.

Cervical. Of the neck.

Clonus. Spasm in which rigidity and relaxation alternate in rapid succession.

Cordotomy. Operation to cut certain pain fibers in the spinal cord, employed mainly in cases of extensive cancer to relieve unbearable pain.

Dendrites. Connections and extensions of a nerve cell which receive impulses and transmit them to the center of the nerve.

Dura mater. Firm connective tissue covering the brain and spinal cord of vertebrates and containing blood vessels.

Electrode gel. A conductive medium providing electrical contact between an electrode surface and the skin.

Epidural electronic stimulation. A technique ₋o propagate electric energy in the region of the spinal cord but not penetrating the dura.

Gate theory of Melzack-Wall. The hypothesis that a neural mechanism in the dorsal horns of the spinal cord acts like a gate which can increase or decrease the flow to the central nervous system.

Hyperalgesia. Extreme sensitivity to pain.

Hypertonic. Muscles stiff; movements awkward.

Intractable pain. Pain which does not respond to conventional methods of treatment.

Myotome. The muscle group innervated by a single spinal nerve.

Nerve root. That part of the nerve as it leaves the spinal cord.

Neuroaugmentive devices. Devices to provide pain relief by blocking the pain signals to the brain.

Paraplegia. Paralysis of the legs and lower part of the body.

Percutanous. Through the skin.

Quadriplegia. Paralysis of all four limbs.

Scoliosis. Lateral curvature of the spine.

Spasticity. An increase over the normal muscle tension associated frequently with clonus and a partial or complete loss of voluntary control.

Subcutanous. Beneath the skin.

TENS. Transcutaneous electrical nerve stimulation.

Transcutaneous. Across the skin.

TERMS RELATED TO THE SKELETON

Appendicular skeleton. Pectoral and pelvic girdles and the limbs.

Ankylosis. Immobility of a joint.

Arthrodesis. Surgical fixation of a joint.

Arthroplasty. Plastic surgery of the joints; formation of movable joints.

Axial skeleton. Skull, vertebral column, ribs and sternum.

Bone cement. Substance which acts solely as a mechanical bond between surface irregularities of different parts eg: a joint prosthesis and the adjacent bone. Considerable bulk of cement is required between the surfaces. (An adhesive is involved in a chemical or physico-chemical interaction between accurately fitted surfaces).

Condyle. A rounded knuckle-like projection on a bone.

Hypertrophic Arthritis. Chronic, morbid enlargement of bone and cartilage occurring chiefly in old people.

Interosseous. Between bones.

Luxation. Dislocation.

Medullary. Marrow or innermost.

Metaphysis. Wide part at the extremity of a long bone.

Osteoarthritis. Chronic multiple degenerative joint disease.

Osteotomy. The surgical cutting of a bone.

Periostium. Dense connective tissue containing blood vessels and covering all bones of the body. An inner layer is composed of a network of thin elastic fibers.

Polycentric. Rotating around more than one center.

Subluxation. Partial dislocation.

Valgus. An adjective denoting a deformity in which a part is bent or twisted outward from the midline of the body.

Index

Acetabulum cup, 26, 32
Acrylic bone cement, 4, 29
Acupuncture, 170
Aesthetic surgery, 148
Anatomy of the ear, 134
Anatomy of the eye, 120
Anatomy of the larynx, 141
Ankle prostheses, 43
Arthritis, 27
Artificial blood, 6
Artificial heart, 68
Artificial kidney, 95
Artificial sphincter, 103
Ascites shunt, 187
Atrial pacemaker lead, 90
Attachment of pacemaker electrodes, 85–92
Attachment of prostheses, 29, 30, 32
A-V sequential demand pacemaker, 81
A-V synchronous pacemaker, 79
Avcothane, 10
Axons, 170

Ball heart valves, 54, 55
Bi-leaflet heart valve, 59
Bilumen mammary implants, 161
Bioglass, 18
Bion, 10
Bioprosthetic heart valves, 61
Biotesting of implant materials, 19–22
Bipolar pacemaker leads, 84
Bjork-Shiley heart valve, 57, 58, 66
Bladder stimulation, 179
Blood, artificial, 6
Blow-out fracture of the orbital floor, 132
Bone, 24, 25
Bone cement, 29
Bone growth stimulation, 45, 183
Bone marrow, 24

Breast augmentation, 14–9
Breast reconstruction after mastectomy, 162
Bubble oxygenator, 51, 52

Caged ball heart valve, 53–56
Caged disc heart valve, 55
Cancellous tissue, 24
Carbon, 11
Carbon fiber—polytetrafluorethylene
    composite, 15
Carbon fiber reinforced carbon, 13
Carbon fiber reinforced UHMWP, 13, 28
Carbon fibers, 10
Cardiovascular circulation, 49
Cardiovascular implants, 48
Cataracts, 121
Central nervous system, 169
Ceramics, 18, 30, 31
Ceravital, 19
Cerebellar electrodes, 181, 183
Cerebellar stimulation, 180
Cerebral palsy, 170
Chest wall defect, 161
Chin augmentation, 148
Chin implant, 150
Chronic pain control, 171
Circumareolar incision, 156
Cobalt-chromium alloys, 17
Cochlear electrical stimulation, 139–140
Cochlear prosthesis, 135–139
Coefficient of friction of joints, 27
Collagen, 15, 24, 149
Composite materials, 13
Condom catheter attachment, 103
Conduction system of the heart, 74
Contact lens, 121
Contour defects, 161
Coonrad total elbow, 35

Correction of ventricular fibrilation, 93
Cosmetic surgery, 148
Crack growth, 24
Cranial defects, 18, 148
Cumulative toxicity index, 21, 22
Custom contoured implants, 161

Deep brain stimulation, 174
Demand pacemaker, 79
Diabetes and impotency, 108
Dialysis, 95
Dialyzation unit, 99
Diaphragm pacing system, 176
Dimethylpolysiloxane, 8
Diploplia, 132
Dorsal column stimulation, 173
Drug release capsules, 10

Ear, 133
ECG, 74
Elbow prosthesis, 34
Elbow structure, 35
Electrocardiogram (ECG), 74
Electrode fixation, 85–92
Electronic diaphragm pacing, 176
Electronic neurostimulation, 168
Electronic stimulation of bone growth, 45
Electronic stimulation of cerebellum, 168
Electronic stimulation of cochlear nerve
    fibers, 135
Electronic stimulation of visual cortex, 170
Electrotherapy, 171
Epicardial implantation of pacemaker
    electrodes, 84, 91
Epilepsy, 180
Erectile elements of the penis, 109, 110
Eustachian tube, 135
External Prosthesis, 44
Extracapsular cataract extraction, 123
Extract tests, 20
Eye, 120

Facial deformities, 148
Facial palsy, 152
Femur, 24
Fibrocystic disease of the breasts, 162
Finger prosthesis, 37

Fixation. *See* Prosthesis fixation
Flexible rod penile implant, 110
Fluosol-DA, 6

Gel-saline mammary implants, 156, 161
Glass-ceramic, 19
Glycine, 15
Gore-Tex vascular grafts, 6

Hall-Kaster heart valve, 59
Hamas total wrist, 36
Heart block, 75
Heart conduction system, 74
Heart lung machine, 48
Heart pacemaker leads, 84
Heart pacemakers, 73
Heart valve fixation, 66
Heart valve prostheses, 53
Hemodialysis, 95
Hemolysis test, 20
Hip prosthesis, 27
Hollow fiber dialyzer, 99
Hydraulic incontinent prosthesis, 103
Hydrocephalus shunt, 184
Hydroxyapatite, 13, 19, 24
Hydroxyproline, 15
Hypertension and impotency, 108
Hypothermia, 51

Impotence, 107
Incontinence, 102
Inflatable mammary prostheses, 157
Inflatable penile implant, 112
Inframammary incision, 153
Intestinal diversion conduit, 102
Intraaortic balloon pump, 10
Intracutaneous injection in rabbits, 20
Intraocular lens, 122
Intravenous lead, 8
Ionescu-Shiley heart valve, 65
Iris, 120

Joints, 26

Kidney, 95
Knee prostheses, 32

Larynx, 141
Left ventricular assist device, 68
Lens implants, 122
Lithium cell powered pacemakers, 77
Loosening of prosthetic joint, 29
Low back pain, 171
Low profile valves, 56
LTI. *See* pyrolitic carbon
Lucite, 4
LVAD, 69

Magovern-Cromie heart valve, 66
Mammary prostheses, 149
Membrane oxygenator, 51
Mercury cell powered pacemakers, 77, 78
Metals, 16
Micturation reflex, 179
Middle ear implants, 135
Modified radical mastectomy, 165
Muscle prosthesis, 45
Myofibroblasts, 156

Nasal strut, 151
Nerve cuff, 175
Neurons, 170
Neurostimulation for the paralyzed bladder, 179
Noninvasive pacemaker programming, 82
Nuclear powered pacemakers, 77

Open heart surgery, 48–50
Orbital floor implants, 132
Orthotic attachment implant, 44
Ossicular replacement prostheses, 135
Ossof-Sisson surgical stent, 143
Otologic implants, 137
Oxygenator, 49, 51

Pacemaker lead attachment, 85–92
Pacemaker leads, 84
Pacemaker programmer, 82
Pacemakers, 73
Patella, 33
Pectoralis muscle implant, 161
Penile implants, 110
Penile reconstruction, 117

Penile sheath, 114
Perfluorodecalin, 6
Peripheral Nerve stimulation, 175
Phaco-emulsifier-aspirator, 123–126
Phantom limb pain, 171
Phrenic nerve stimulation, 177
"Piggy-back" mammary prosthesis, 165
Pivotal disc heart valve, 62
Platinum 18, 77
Plexiglas, 4
Polyester, 7
Polyethylene, 1, 5
Poly-2-hydroxyethyl methacrylate, 5
Polymeric carbon, 11
Polymers, 1
Polymethyl methacrylate, 4
Polyolefin elastomer, 10, 38
Polysulfone, 7
Polytetrafluoroethylene, 5
Polyurethane, 8, 91
Porous materials, 5, 6, 7, 88
Portable dialysis system, 97
Proline, 15
Properties of implant materials, 3
Proplast, 15
Prosthesis fixation, 29, 30, 44, 58, 85, 104, 133
Prosthetic heart, 68
Prosthetic heart valves, 53
Protasul, 17
Psychogenic impotence, 108
PTFE, 5
Ptotic breasts, 159
Pyrolite, 12
Pyrolitic carbon, 12

Rabbit muscle implant test, 20
Reconstruction after mastectomy, 162
Recovery of spermatazoa, 104
Regional vasodilation, 174
Respiratory paralysis, 176
Retina, 120
Rhinoplasty implant, 149

Saddle joint, 26
Safety of implant materials, 19
Shoulder prosthesis, 39
Silicon nitride, 19

Silicone copolymer, 10
Silicone mammary prostheses, 149
Silicone rubber, 9, 36, 143, 148
Silicone rubber joints, 36
Silicones, 8
Skeleton, 24
Spermatocele implant, 104
Spinal cord stimulator,
Stainless steel, 17
Stapendectomy prosthesis, 137
Stents, 102, 118
Stimulation of peripheral nerves, 175
Stroma, 104
Subcutaneous mastectomy, 163
Sutureless pacemaker electrode, 92
Synovial membrane, 27
Systemic toxicity in mice, 21

Talar component, 43
Tantalum, 18
Tendon prosthesis, 45
TENS, 171
Testicular implants, 116
Thermoplastic polymers, 2
Thermosetting polymers, 2
Tilting disc heart valve, 57, 59
Tissue culture test, 19, 20, 21
Titanium, 16
Tivanium, 16
Toe prostheses, 43
Total artificial heart, 68
Total penile reconstruction, 117
Toxicological testing, 19

Transaxillary incision, 157
Transcutaneous electrical nerve stimulation, 171
Transvenous implantation of pacemaker leads, 76, 84
Tympanic membrane, 134
Tympanostomy ventilation tubes, 138

ULTI. See pyrolitic carbon
Ultra-high molecular weight polyethylene (UHMWP), 5
Ultra-low temperature isotropic carbon, 13
Unipolar pacemaker leads, 84
Ureteral stent, 101
Urinary incontinence prosthesis, 102

Vaginal stent, 118
Valves, 53
Vascular prostheses, 70
Ventricular fibrilation, 93
Visual cortex, 121
Vitallium, 17
Vitreous carbon, 12
Voice Prosthesis, 145
Voice restoration, 141
Volz total elbow, 35

Wearable artifical kidney, 95
Wrist prosthesis, 36

Xenograft heart valves, 63